GASTRIC BAND HYPNOSIS

Proven Hypnosis to Lose Weight and Transform Your Body. Control Sugar Cravings and Food Addiction with Guided Meditations for Rapid, Massive and Lasting Weight Loss

CAROLINE LEAN

© Copyright 2020 - All rights reserved.

Table of Contents

Introduction

I f you think you will be happy when you reach your ideal weight but get stuck on a negative view of your body, it will not work.

Have you noticed that when you get up on the wrong foot, you are all day in a bad mood, and you think that the spell is going on because you only get nasty things? On the contrary, with a cheerful mood, people seem more pleasant to you, smiling, you feel light.

You have unknowingly emitted a vibration towards the universe, which sends your thoughts back to you. The positive attracts the positive. The negative brings you a negative result. This form of energy is transmitted to the universe, and it influences what you will get from your unconscious request. Above all, do not focus on everything negative about weight, calories, fat, diet, suffering in an intensive sports practice. You just attract them with thought. On the other hand, if you focus on the result you want to achieve, if you see this evolution step by step, you will modify your lifestyle to make this positive result for you.

How can positive thinking be the most powerful solution for programming our brain and dictating that it make us lose weight easily?

Demons, get out of our heads!

These demons (ideas, beliefs, emotions) build what we are by very powerful influence, the law of coherence. The obsessive desire to be and to appear consistent in our behavior sometimes pushes us to act contrary to our interests.

In other words, unconscious pressures force us to react to agree with what we choose to believe. This self-persuasion applies in all choices, and it is impossible for us that our opinions are different from what we have already decided, even if it means lying to us from time to time.

So choosing to think every day that one is overweight unconsciously leads to doing what it takes to be!

So, high resolution, we are going to start losing weight by diet or any other method!

Yes, but, as soon as we start to feel lighter, the brain panics because it is not consistent with the image of the choice that our mind makes daily (the fact that we think we are overweight).

That is when our demons come to tug us. "I feel better slimmer, but, strangely, I am pushed to crack and eat anything to feel better." Personally, the speech of my mind to allow me to make a gap (a big gap of sugar in general), was "you have made efforts, you can have fun, you will take things back seriously after." It was a big lie to return to an image consistent with my misconceptions about my physique.

Without understanding that the method we are choosing is not the right solution, we blame ourselves for not having succeeded. The snacking trend is reinstalling, and so is the yo-yo. Making positive affirmations means talking to yourself aloud (preferably when you are alone!). By telling yourself positive words, considering the incredible results, it doesn't cost anything to try!

It is a method of personal development that is used to reprogram your brain to think positively. You can make positive statements for your health, your work or your self-confidence, your relationships, etc.

The goal is to attract happiness by pronouncing it! At first, one does not believe frankly in what one says. The lyrics are even the opposite of what we think, but by dint of saying it, the brain will believe it, and so will we! That is how they will have a real impact on our lives.

CHAPTER 1:

Concepts of Hypnosis

The hypnotic stomach band operates in all the same means as the physical one: your consumption of food is limited by your body to make sure that you feel delighted after minimal dishes. There are simply three vital distinctions between the physical and also the hypnotic band.

1. With a hypnotic band, all modifications are instantly done by proceeding to use the hypnotic trance.

2. With the hypnotic band, there is no physical surgical procedure, and for this reason, no physical threats.

3. The hypnotic band is numerous hundreds of bucks less expensive.

What Happens to Your Body during Hypnosis?

How do you recognize when you have had adequate to consume? Initially, you can feel the weight as well as the area of the food. When your tummy is complete, the food presses versus and also extends the tummy wall surface, as well as the nerve endings in the tummy wall surface, respond. As we saw in Phase 2, when these nerves are promoted, they send out a signal to the mind to obtain the sensation, "I have had sufficient."

Second of all, as the belly fills out and also food gets in the intestinal tract, PYY, as well as GLP-1, is launched and set off a feeling of complete satisfaction in the mind that likewise motivates us to quit consuming.

However, when individuals persistently eat way too much, they end up being desensitized to both the anxious signals and also the same neuropeptide signaling system. Throughout the setup hypnotic trance, we make use of hypnotherapy and even images to resensitize the mind to these signals. Your hypnotic band improves the full effect of these worried as well as neuropeptide messages.

With the benefit of hypnotherapy, we can alter this system and also enhance your level of sensitivity to these signals, to make sure that you feel completely satisfied as quickly as you have consumed sufficient to fill up that tiny bag on top of your tummy.

A hypnotic stomach band makes your body act precisely as though you have gone through the surgery. It restricts your belly as well as modifies the signals from your belly to your mind, so you feel complete swiftly.

The hypnotic band uses several amazing features of hypnotherapy. The hypnotherapy enables us to speak straight to parts of the mind and body that are not under mindful control. Extraordinary as it might appear, in hypnotherapy, we can encourage the body to act in different ways even though our mindful mind has no methods of routing that adjustment.

The Power of Hypnotherapy

There are many more instances of just how the mind can straight and impact the body. We understand that persistent tension can trigger tummy abscess, and also an emotional shock can transform somebody's hair grey overnight. Nonetheless, what I specifically like regarding hypnotherapy treatment is just how the mind impacts the body in a favorable and also restorative mean.

The human being wonders that ideas, as well as hypnotherapy, can trigger extensive physical modifications in your body.

Hypnotic trance, all on its own, has an obvious physical result. One of the most instant results is that topics discover it deeply loosening up. Remarkably, one of the most frequent monitoring that my customers report after I have seen them—despite what we have been working with—is that their family and friends tell them they look more youthful.

Cybernetic Loophole

Your mind, as well as body, remains in regular interaction in a cybernetic loophole: they regularly affect each other as the mind unwinds in hypnotherapy, so as well does the body. When the body unwinds, it really feels far better, and also it sends out that message to the mind, which subsequently really feels far better and unwinds additionally. This procedure minimizes anxiety and also makes much more power readily available to the recovery and even the body's immune systems.

The therapeutic impacts of hypnotherapy do not need hoax or memory loss. The enzymes that generate swelling are not launched. Also, because of this, the melt does not advance to a higher degree of damages, and also there is marginal discomfort throughout recovery.

By utilizing hypnotherapy and also visualization, our bodies make points that are entirely outside their conscious control. Self-control will not make these types of modifications, yet creativity is more powerful than the will. By utilizing hypnotherapy and visualization to chat straight to the subconscious mind, we can make a physical distinction in as low as 20 mins.

With hypnotherapy, we can significantly boost the impact of the mind upon the body. When we fit your hypnotic stomach band, we are using specifically the very same system of hypnotic interaction to the subconscious mind. We connect to the mind with dazzling images. Also, the mind changes your body's responses, improving your physical response to food to make sure that your belly is tightened, and so you feel truly complete after merely a couple of mouthfuls.

What Makes the Hypnotherapy Job So Well?

Some individuals discover it unsubstantiated that hypnotherapy, as well as images, can have such a severe and also effective result.

In some cases, the skeptic and the client, coincide individual. We desire the outcomes, yet we battle to think that it truly will function. At the awareness degree, our minds are aware of the distinction between what we visualize along with physical facts. Nevertheless, one more incredible hypnotic sensation shows that no matter what, our company believes at the mindful degree since hypnotherapy permits our mind to reply to a truth that is entirely independent of what we knowingly assume. This sensation is called "hypnotic trance reasoning."

It is feasible to be hypnotized and also have a hypnotic stomach band fitted and yet to "recognize" with your aware mind that you do not have medical marks as well as you do not have a physical stomach band placed. Hypnotic trance reasoning suggests that part of your mind can think one point, along with one more component, can think the full reverse, and also your body and mind can continue functioning, thinking two various points hold. So you will undoubtedly be able knowingly to understand that you have not paid hundreds of bucks for surgery, and yet at the innermost degree of subconscious command, your body thinks that you have a stomach band as well as will certainly act as necessary. Consequently, your tummy is promoted to indicate "really feeling complete" to your mind after merely a couple of mouthfuls of food. So you feel completely satisfied while you slim down.

How Effective Is Hypnotherapy?

The hypnotherapy we utilize to produce your stomach band utilizes "visualization" and "affect-laden images." Visualization is merely the production of images in your mind. We can all do it. It becomes part of the reasoning. For instance, think about your front door and ask on your own which side the lock gets on. To respond to that concern, you see an image in your mind's eye. It does not matter in any way just how sensible or intense the picture is; it is merely the method your mind functions, and also you view as high as you require to see.

Affect-laden images are the emotional term for psychologically significant photos. In this procedure, we make use of images of psychological's eye that have psychological value. Although hypnotic pointers are useful, they are drastically improved by helpful photos when we are connecting straight to the body. For instance, you might not have the ability to accelerate your heart by merely informing it to defeat quicker. Yet, if you picture basing on a train line as well as seeing a train hurrying in the direction of you, your heart quickens quite swiftly. Your body reacts extremely incredibly to vibrant, purposeful photos.

That is why I will certainly explain your procedure in the hypnotic trance area. It doesn't matter whether you are paying attention purposely; your subconscious mind will undoubtedly listen to all it requires to duplicate the genuine band, in all the same manner in which a dazzling photo of a coming close to train impacts your heart price.

You do not require to hold the images of the functional treatments in your aware mind; as a result of the program throughout a procedure, you are anesthetized and also subconscious. Despite what you knowingly keep in mind, under the hypnotic anesthetic, your subconscious mind utilizes all this info, and even images to mount your stomach band is precisely the appropriate location.

The Power of Context

Contextual signs are one more considerable element of the hypnotic pointer. As an example, when I did my hypnotic performance, the context of the theater, the lights, the stage, and the assumptions of the target market all boosted the hypnotic sensations, despite whether the individuals were knowingly familiar with it.

The same holds with the stomach band. I described in the last phase the prep work that cosmetic surgeons need before the physical stomach band procedure, also, you must adhere to the very same primary treatment too. That will reproduce the physical context for the procedure within your very own body. That makes it easier for hypnotherapy to have an immediate, effective result and also installed the modifications you require to create right into your body.

The doctors ask their people to stroll at the very least 20 mins a day. If you build up all the strolling, you perform in a day, and mostly all people currently do this. Just a few non-active individuals stroll less than this. Nonetheless, if you desire, you can make sure you do it by challenging taking a specific stroll of thirty minutes, as an example by strolling to the following bus quit or to the regional park and also go back. The factor of the strolling is not health and fitness or workout, yet only making sure excellent blood flows in the legs. When you do it, your prep work for your hypnotic stomach band corresponds to the prep work for a medical stomach band.

A silver lining impact, nonetheless, is that it will certainly establish you up for the workout that your body will certainly intend to do when you reduce weight. This might appear strange to you currently, however, as you reach your all-natural healthy and balanced weight, you will undoubtedly turn into one of those individuals that are generally slim, in shape and also really appreciate strolling as well as numerous various other kinds of workout.

CHAPTER 2:

Hypnosis and Weight Loss

Even if hypnosis has no physical side effects, for it to be effective, it has to be done well and by a certified hypnotist. There are many hypnotists in the market, but getting the right one is a challenge. We shall give you a guide into getting an excellent hypnotist to help in your weight loss journey. We shall also discuss various apps that use hypnosis to aid in weight loss as well as a guide to losing weight through hypnotherapy.

Choosing a Hypnotherapist for Weight Loss

Expanding open, GP, and NHS acknowledgment of necessary treatments, hypnotherapy has explicitly brought about a gigantic increment in the number of individuals offering to prepare. The nature of this preparation fluctuates incredibly, so it is the BSCH's (British Society of Clinical Hypnosis) main goal to give its specialists an abnormal state of preparing and moral practice.

There are various things you are encouraged to search for when searching for a trance inducer to assist you with a specific issue:

- Where was the preparation for them?

- Have they passed an independent audit?

- Do you have academic validity in your preparation?

- Is there a continuous preparing framework or a CPD framework?

- Is there a supervisory framework?

- Do they have protection for expert remuneration?

- Do they pursue a composed morals code?

- Is there a formal grumbling strategy for them?

- Are they individuals from an expert body broadly perceived?

- Can you call an inquiry or grievance to that body?

All BSCH individuals are prepared in high quality. We set particular requirements for experts of hypnotherapy. Inside the online database, you will discover various sorts of participation as laid out underneath all can, in any event, a decent degree of expertise.

- **Associate Member**—qualified trance specialist with a go from a perceived preparing school at the diploma/PG Cert level.

- **Full Member**—qualified trance specialist with a go off in any event diploma/PG Cert level from a perceived school of preparing and extra authorize master preparing (for example, a practitioner or cognitive behavioral level pass).

- **Diplomat**—as a full part, however, on an essential clinical subject with an acknowledged paper.

- **Fellow**—full or diplomatic part moved up to extraordinary administration or accomplishment from inside the general public.

The different accompanying tips will manage you all the while:

Get a referral for yourself. Ask somebody you trust, similar to a companion or relative, if they have been to a trance inducer or on the off chance that they know somebody they has.

1. **Ask for a referral from a qualified organization.** A certified subliminal specialist might be prescribed by your PCP, chiropractor, analyst, dental specialist, or another therapeutic expert. They will likewise work with some information of your medicinal history that can enable them to prescribe a specific trance specialist in your condition.

2. **Search online for a subliminal specialist.** The Register of General Hypnotherapy and the American Clinical Hypnosis Society are phenomenal areas to start an inquiry. Visit roughly about six sites. A private site of trance inducers can offer you a smart thought of what they resemble, regardless of whether they explicitly spend significant time in anything and give some understanding into their systems and foundation. Check to see whether earlier patients have tributes. Ensure the site records the certifications of the trance inducers.

3. **Check the protection with you.** On the off chance that you have psychological well-being protection, you can call them. You can likewise get to this information on the site of your insurance agencies. Call your state mental affiliation or state guiding affiliation and ask for the names of confirmed clinicians or approved master advisors who rundown entrancing as one of their strengths.

4. **If required, think about a long-separation arrangement.** Quality over solace is consistently the best approach with regards to your well-being, on the off chance that in your quick district you experience issues finding a gifted trance inducer, extend your inquiry

span to incorporate other neighboring urban communities or neighborhoods.

5. **Ask for accreditation.** No confirmed projects are gaining practical experience in hypnotherapy at noteworthy colleges. Instead, numerous trance specialists have degrees in different regions, for example, drug, dentistry, or advising, and have experienced additional hypnotherapy preparing.

6. Check for training in different fields, for example, medication, brain research, or social work.

7. **Be cautious about the so-called hypnotherapy specialists.** They may have gotten their doctorate from an unaccredited college on the off chance that they don't have a degree in another restorative segment.

8. A believable and proficient trance specialist will have proficient offices, inside and out entrancing information, and evidence of the accomplishment of past clients.

9. Check whether the specialist is part of an association.

10. **Match the specialization of a therapist with your prerequisites.** Hypnotherapy can be a viable pressure and tension treatment. It can likewise profit interminable agony sufferers, hot flashes, and successive migraines. Most advisors will list their strengths on their sites. However, you ought to also inquire as to whether they have any experience managing your particular side effects. On the off chance that you have eternal back agony, for example, endeavor to discover a trance specialist who is likewise a chiropractor or general expert.

11. Ask numerous inquiries. You offer the specialist a chance to find out about you as such.

You will likewise have a sentiment of how well the subliminal specialist can tune in to your prerequisites.

    a. How long have they been prepared?

    b. How long have they drilled?

    c. The specialist should have the option to explain the differentiation between things, for example, formal and casual stupor and what awareness levels are.

12. **Say the discoveries you are searching for to the specialist.** A unique treatment plan ought to be imparted to you by the trance specialist dependent on your manifestations. Be apparent about what you plan to achieve. "I need to shed pounds" or "I need to kill ceaseless joint torment." You ought to likewise be posed inquiries about your medicinal history or any past hypnotherapy experience.

    a. Make sure that the trance specialist invites you.

    b. Was the workplace spotless and amicable with the staff?

    c. To ensure you locate the correct fit, go on a couple of discussions.

13. **Finding a trance inducer, trust your premonitions.** At that point, feel free to arrange the event that you feel energetic or extraordinary about proceeding. Ensure you know and feel great with their methodology. Get some information about rates or costs and what number of visits your concern typically requires.

14. **Consider pricing around.** Now and then, insurance covers hypnotherapy. However, it contrasts. Check your arrangement to ensure you make an arrangement. If your insurance secures it, copayments can extend from $30 to $50 per visit. A subliminal specialist arrangement could cost $50 to $275 without insurance.

Best Hypnotic Weight Loss Apps

1. **Learning Self Hypnosis by Patrick Browning.** That is a superb application to unwind following a protracted day at employment! I appreciate merely utilizing it for 30 minutes to take a portion of my day by day weight. Of note is that all that you need to do in the application costs additional money.

2. **Digipill.** Digipill enables you to tackle your rest issue and unwind! It is additionally a precise instrument for helping you to get in shape, gain certainty, and significantly more!

3. **Health and Fitness with Hypnosis, Meditation, and Music.** With this basic, however amazing application, you can get fit rapidly and keep sound. It is a helpful device that enables individuals to shed pounds by utilizing trance.

4. **Harmony.** Amicability is a simple method to think and unwind! You can decrease tension with this free instrument, acquire certainty, and significantly more!

5. **Free Hypnosis.** It is a basic, however, fantastic asset for simple unwinding that contains valuable strategies and activities!

6. **Stress Relief Hypnosis: Anxiety, Relax, and Sleep.** For those battling with sleep deprivation and nervousness, this free instrument is flawless.

Step by Step Guide to Hypnotherapy for Weight Loss

1. **Believe.** If you don't figure entrancing will enable you to change your emotions, it's probably going to have little impact.

2. **Become agreeable.** Go to a spot where you may not be stressed. That can resemble your bed, a couch, or an agreeable, comfortable chair anyplace. Ensure you bolster your head and neck. Wear loose

garments and ensure the temperature is set at an agreeable level. It might be simpler to unwind if you play some delicate, particularly something instrumental.

3. **Focus on an item.** Discover something to take a gander at and focus on in the room, ideally something somewhat above you. Utilize your concentration for clearing your leader of all contemplations on this item. Make this article the main thing that you know.

4. **Breathing is crucial.** When you close your eyes, inhale profoundly. Reveal to yourself the greatness of your eyelids and let them fall delicately. Inhale profoundly with an ordinary mood as your eyes close. Concentrate on your breathing, enabling it to assume control over your whole personality, much the same as the item you've been taking a gander at previously. Feel progressively loose with each fresh breath. Envision that your muscles disperse all the pressure and stress. Permit this inclination from your face, your chest, your arms, lastly, your legs to descend your body. When you're entirely loose, your psyche ought to be precise.

5. **Display a pendulum.** Customarily, the development of a pendulum moving to and fro has been utilized to energize the center. Picture this pendulum in your psyche, moving to and fro. Concentrate on it as you unwind to help clear your brain.

6. **Start by focusing from 10 to 1 in your mind.** You advise yourself as you check down that you are steadily getting further into entrancing. State, "10. I'm alleviating. 9. I get increasingly loose. 8. I can feel my body spreading unwinding. 7. Nothing yet unwinding I can feel... 1. I'm resting profoundly."

7. **Waking up from self-hypnosis.** You have accomplished what you need, and you should wake up. From 1 to 10, check back. State in your mind: "1. I wake up. 2. I'll feel like I woke up from a significant

rest when I tally down. 3. I feel wakeful more... 10. I'm wakeful, and I'm new."

8. **Develop a plan.** You ought to endeavor in a condition of holding yourself ultimately to go through around twenty minutes per day. While beneath, shift back and forth between portions of the underneath referenced methodologies. Attempt to assault your poor eating rehearses from any edge.

Learn to refrain from emotional overeating. You are not intrigued by the frightful nibble of food you experience.

CHAPTER 3:

Experience of Losing Weight with Hypnosis

Wanted to lose weight and sustain it with hypnosis? You can use the therapist's suggestions long-term. Many patients report that after hypnosis, they were convinced that, for example, fatty foods do not taste good, water tastes better than lemonade, or fruit and vegetables are delicious. The suggestions made in hypnosis make renunciation very easy because it is no longer perceived as negative.

For one to achieve success depends on whether the person concerned is ready for changes, for example, in eating habits. Dieting is also advisable to support hypnosis. However, hypnosis makes it much easier to overcome negative habits and behavior patterns and to establish positive ones, thus, make losing weight a success. Therefore, many more people are successful in losing weight with hypnosis than without this tool.

Step-By-Step Self-Hypnosis for Weight Loss

Hypnosis is an excellent tool that can change your life, just as we have said earlier. I think it's a tool that deserves recognition because most people don't know how to use their brains. That is something that you, unfortunately, do not learn in the school system.

The goal is to act on the automatisms that you do not control by will. If tomorrow I tell you to lose weight all by yourself or to stop having food compulsions, you are going to tell me that you cannot do it because you do not control anything. It is "stronger than you" to power this mechanism without wanting to.

My role is, therefore, to act on your memory, to act on the unconscious automatisms, in other words, program your brain in such a way that it loses weight without you knowing and surprise you to lose weight quickly. That sounds great, right? By doing diets in general, we send the body the message that it is not able to regulate itself by itself and believed for a long time that you had to control with your mind the way you eat, but it doesn't work like that; you did not ask yourself all these questions; it was your body that acted for you. That is also why parents always said: "Finish your plates," "Children don't starve, you must eat," "Eat if you want to grow." However, as a child, you knew your needs perfectly and your limits without anybody having to make you aware of what you needed.

You have to help your body to find its place so that it can regulate itself by itself and make you lose weight easily without thinking about it.

You should also look for the trigger for your weight gain because as long as we have not acted on it, you will continue to loop forever.

Your unconscious is a fabulous reservoir of resources that records all your learning since your birth. When you learned to walk, for example, you fell about two thousand times before you managed to balance. Yet today, you are not aware of walking. It is entirely reasonable—you imprinted this process in your memory without knowing it.

That is the reason why my goal is to accompany your unconscious towards "another thing to do" so that you can slim down easily and sustain success. Take time to know how self-hypnosis works.

Self-hypnosis is getting the brain used to a specific pattern, preparing it in advance because the unconscious will facilitate progress towards something it knows. So, it is better to accustom this part of the brain to something positive—to success—rather than to a disaster. To succeed, you have to do it the right way, and this can be a real boost, especially for weight-related issues.

Addressing Your Unconscious

To start, we will have to define its goal; it is objective. We will, therefore, take the time to list the reasons that push us to make this change by asking the right questions: What do I want? Does it depend only on me? Why is it important to me? What will it bring me? We'll formulate the objective to be achieved by a sentence that we will repeat. Be careful, however, that we do not speak to the unconscious as to anyone. For a good reason, our unconscious remains at seven years of mental age and does not understand specific formulations—for example, negation; when we repeat "I mustn't eat," the only thing the brain hears is "eat."

So, choose your words carefully; you will use a somewhat positive message. We often talk about "losing weight"; as a reflex, we don't like to lose, so we would rather say "gain in lightness." As an example, we could use the following formulations of objectives: "I reach my healthy weight gradually over time" or "I contribute to my well-being by doing exercises daily and by eating healthy."

The idea is to find a sentence that you can understand, remember, and repeat as often as you want.

Visualize to Prepare

Some studies in mental imagery have shown that having a real experience or merely imagining it animates the same areas in the brain. Visualization will, therefore, have a real impact on the pursuit of the objective. Indeed, the unconscious moves more easily towards what it knows. Bringing the brain to life by imagining it will allow it to reproduce it easier.

Each day, you should take time for viewing.

For more efficiency, we will ritualize the process. We will sit quietly without being disturbed, in a comfortable position, and perhaps even with music. The moments before we fall asleep is the ideal time to practice visualization. Since the brain processes information during sleep, exercising the brain during that time will be more effective.

A useful visualization exercise is that of projecting into the future. We can imagine the whole day going from dawn to bedtime once the objective has been reached. How are we going to behave? What will change? Does this new identity look alike? We have to go into detail and imagine what this day would be equivalent.

Another exercise will be that of fetish clothing. When we have a weight goal, we often have a reference garment that we use as a goal. One can thus, imagine oneself with the garment in question. What reaction does our appearance elicit? What are our feelings?

Finally, we identify an exercise that will satisfy those who are keener on weighing. With an ideal figure to reach, we can very well imagine it appearing on the scale and projecting ourselves into the feeling of satisfaction and success that this could provide us.

You will understand if, in weight loss or weight gain, diet and physical activity are essential; the work of the mind through self-hypnosis can be a real ally and make all the difference!

Practical Steps for Self-Hypnosis to Lose Weight

Processing of losing weight through hypnosis is to program our mind in such a way that it can make and accept a suggestion. During hypnosis, our mind is positioned in such a way that it accesses the depths of its subconscious to eradicate beliefs and to think that can interfere with achieving the desired goal. That makes hypnosis to be popular among those who want to lose weight. However, there may be no reason to seek the services of a professional weight-loss hypnosis trainer if this guide is diligently followed. Most of the insurance plans do not shelter the cost of hypnotherapy. Try to follow the guideline of this self-hypnosis to lose weight.

Step 1

Set a perfect weight loss goal for yourself. Aim for an available amount of weight you want to shield and choose a specific time for which you want to achieve weight loss. Always read your goal out loud before you begin.

Step 2

Always try to view yourself in the body size you want to be. Try to imagine yourself in your dream shape and the ideal weight you have been longing for; also, try to view your friends' and family's reaction when they will see you in that body and what they will say. Make sure you make the scene as lively and positive as much as possible to trigger some colors, fragrance, sounds, and feelings.

Step 3

Relax your whole body while closing your eyes as if you are drowning until you feel your whole body immerse and become completely soft. Continue to breathe for three minutes until you can feel a different sensation running through your body, relaxing all parts of it. You will see yourself in a different state of trance.

Step 4

Imagine seeing your ideal body in that trance. Thinking about how you feel in your new body and experience the world around you—how other people will see you and how you will feel good about being healthy and having a physically fit body. Do this for at least two minutes. Then view your body in a new state of balance.

Step 5

Slowly return your body to your current state. Be very intentional to bring back the feelings of positive inner experience with you. If you continue to do this daily, you will be able to train your body and mind to know how good it is to lose weight. The necessary behavioral changes that your body needs to lose weight.

Repeat this process daily for two months and recheck your weight to know the amount of weight you have lost.

How This Works on Your Body

There is a spot—called the door of dreams—between the right and the left part of the brain. This "balance" manner is a tool that you can use to set up motivation, love, self-esteem, indifference, disgust, shrinking stomach… That's the part that helps you to change how you see yourself and transform you to whatever you believe you are; by using it, you become your hypnotist, and session after a session; you will lose weight.

Some hypnotists, but still few, know how to induce a hypnotic trance deep enough to be able to establish motivation, love, self-esteem, indifference, disgust, stomach shrinking in their clients. Also, many other techniques specific to hypnotists allow their clients to lose weight. So, this is why you need to take the self-hypnosis teaching seriously.

You can—and it will undoubtedly happen to you—fall asleep during a session of self-hypnosis; it is either because you are exhausted and your brain does not have the strength to concentrate, or you are motivated. You start dreaming and fall asleep, or the session is too long, and your brain must fall asleep to recharge.

CHAPTER 4:

Mindful Eating Habits

Take Things Slowly

Eating should not be treated as a race. Eat slowly. This just means that you should take your time to relish and enjoy your food—it's a healthy thing! So, how long do you have to grind up the food in your mouth? Well, there is no specific time food should be chewed, but 18-25 bites are enough to enjoy the food mindfully. This can be hard at first, mainly if you have been used to speed eating for a very long time.

Why not try some different techniques like using chopsticks when you are accustomed to spoon and fork? Or use your non-dominant hand when eating. These strategies can slow you down and improve your awareness.

Avoid Distractions

To make things simpler for you, just make it a habit of sitting down and staying away from distractions. The handful of nuts that you eat as you walk through the kitchen and the bunch of morning snacks you nibbled while standing in front of your fridge can be hard to recall. According to researchers, people tend to eat more when they are doing other things too. You should, therefore, sit down and focus on your food to prevent mindless eating behaviors.

Savor Every Bite

Do not forget that eating is not only about enjoying the food you eat, but your health too, and without feeling guilty and uncomfortable. Relishing the sight, taste, and smell of your diet is indeed worth it. This can be so easy if you take things gradually and don't rush to perfection. Make small changes towards awareness until you are a fully mindful eater. So, eat slowly and savor the good food you are eating and the proper nutrition you are giving to your body.

Mind the Presentation

Regardless of how busy you are, it is a good idea to set the table—making sure it looks divine. A lovely set of utensils, placement, and napkin made of eco-friendly cloth material is a perfect reminder that you need to sit down and pay attention when you have your meals.

Plate Your Food

Serving yourself and portioning your food before you bring the plate to the table can help you to consume a modest amount, rather than putting a platter on the table from which to replenish continually. You can do this even with crackers, chips, nuts, and other snack foods. Keep yourself away from the temptation of eating straight from a bag of chips and different types of food. It is also helpful if you resize the bag or place the food in smaller containers so that you can stay conscious of the amount of food you are eating. Having a bright idea of how much you have eaten will make you stop eating when you're full, or even sooner.

Always Choose Quality over Quantity

By trying to select smaller amounts of the most beautiful food within your means, you will end up enjoying and feeling satisfied without the chance of overeating. With this, it will be helpful if you spend time preparing your meals using quality and fresh ingredients. Cooking can be a relaxing and pleasurable experience if you only let yourself into it. On top of this, you can achieve the peace of mind that comes from knowing what is in the food you are eating.

Don't Invite Your Thoughts and Emotions to Dinner

Just as there are many other factors that affect our sense of mindful eating, as well as the digestive system, it would come as no surprise that our thoughts and emotions play just as much of an important role.

It happens on the odd occasion that one comes home after a long and tiresome day, and you feel somewhat "worked up," irritated, and angry. This is when negative and even destructive thoughts creep in while you are having supper.

The best practice would be to avoid this altogether. Therefore, if you are feeling unhappy or angry in any way, go for a walk before supper, play with your children, or play with your family pet. But, whatever you do, take your mind off your negative emotions before you attempt to have a meal.

Make a Good Meal Plan for Each Week

When you start the diet, it is advised to stick to the meal plan that comes with the diet. There should be a meal plan of 2 weeks or four weeks attached to the diet's guideline. Once you are familiar with the food list, prohibited ingredients, cooking techniques, and how to go grocery shopping for your diet, it will be easier for you to twist and change things in the meal plan. Do not try to change the meal plan for the first two weeks. Stick to the meal plan they give you. If you decide to change it right at the beginning, you may feel lost or feel terrified then. So, it is advised to try and introduce new recipes and ideas after you are two weeks into the diet.

Drink Lots of Water

Staying hydrated is vital to living a healthy life in general. It is not relevant for only diets, but in general, we should always be drinking enough water to keep ourselves hydrated. Dehydration can bring forth many unwanted diseases. When you are dehydrated, you feel very dizzy, lightheaded, nauseous, and lethargic. You cannot focus on anything well. Urinary infection occurs, which triggers other health issues.

The purpose of drinking water is to help you process the different food you are eating and to help digest it well. Water helps in proper digestion; it helps in extracting bad minerals from our body. Water also gives us a glow on the skin.

Never Skip Breakfast

It is essential to eat a full breakfast to keep yourself moving actively throughout the day. It gives you a significant boost, proper metabolism, and your digestion starts appropriately functioning during the day. When you skip breakfast, everything sort of disrupts. Your day starts slow, and soon, you would feel restless. It is essential to have a good meal at the beginning of your day in order to be productive for the rest of the day. If you are very busy, try to have your breakfast on the go. Grab breakfast in a box or a mason jar and have it in the car or on the bus or transport of any kind you are using to get to your work. You can also have your breakfast at a healthy restaurant where they serve food that is in sync with your diet.

Eat Protein

Protein is perfect for the body. It helps your brain function better. It can come from both animal and non-animal products. So even if you are a vegetarian or vegan, you can still enjoy your protein from plants. Soy, mushroom, legumes, and nuts are a few examples.

Eating protein keeps you strong and healthy, it increases your brain function. On the contrary, if you do not eat enough protein for the day, your entire way would be wasted. You will not be able to focus on anything properly. You would feel dizzy and weak all through the day. If you are a vegetarian or vegan, you can enjoy avocado, coconut, almond, cashew, soy, and mushroom to get protein.

Eat Super Foods

Most people eat foods that do not necessarily affect them in the best way. Where some foods may enhance some people's energy levels, it may impact others more negatively.

The important thing is to know your food. It may be a good idea to keep a food journal, and if you know that certain foods affect you negatively, one should try to avoid those foods and stick to healthier options.

It is a fact that the majority enjoy foods that they should probably not be eating. However, if you wish to eat mindfully and enhance your health and a general sense of well-being, then it would be best to eat foods that will do precisely that.

There are also various foods that are classified as superfoods. These would include your lean and purest sources of protein, such as free-range chicken, as well as a variety of fresh fruits, vegetables, and herbs.

Stop Multitasking While You Eat

Multitasking is defined as the simultaneous execution of more than one activity at one time. Though it is a skill that we should master, it often leads to unproductive business. The development of our economy leads to a more hectic way of living. Most of us develop the habit of doing one thing while doing another. This is true even when it comes to eating.

Smaller Plates, Taller Glasses

This habit changer ties in a little bit with drinking more water; however, it's a bit different. People tend to fill up their plates with food, so the size of the plate matters. If you have a large plate, you're going to put more food on your plate but, if you have a smaller plate, you will have less food on your plate.

Stay Positive

The secret to succeeding in anything is positive. When you start something new, always stay positive regarding it. You need to keep a positive mind, an open mind rather. You cannot be anxious, hasty, and restless in a diet. You need to stay calm and do everything that calms you down. Overthinking can lead to being bored and not interested in the diet very soon. The power of positivity is immense. It cannot be compared with anything else. On the other hand, when you start something with a negative mindset, it eventually does not work out. You end up leaving it behind or failing at it because you had doubts right at the beginning. A doubtful mind cannot focus properly, and the best never comes out from a doubtful mind.

CHAPTER 5:

Stop Emotional Eating

Emotional eating occurs typically when your food becomes a tool that you use in responding to any internal or external emotional cues. It's normal for human beings to tend to react to any stressful situation and the difficult feelings that they have. Whenever you have stressful emotions, you tend to run after a bag of chips or bars of chocolate, a large pizza, or a jar of ice cream to distract yourself from that emotional pain. The foods that you crave at that moment are referred to as comfort food. Those foods contain a high calorie or high carbohydrate with no nutritional value.

Do you know that your appetite increases whenever you are stressed, and whenever you're stressed, you tend to make poor eating habits? Stress is associated with weight gain and weight loss. When you are under intense pressure and intense emotions like boredom or sadness, you tend to cleave unto food. Now that's emotion napping, and it is the way that your body relieves itself of the stress and gets the energy that it needs to overcome its over-dependence on food. Usually get you to the point whereby you don't eat healthy anymore.

Emotional eating is a chronic issue that affects every gender, both male and female, but research has shown that women are more prone to emotional eating than men. Emotional eaters tend to incline towards salty, sweet, fatty, and generally high-calorie foods. Usually, these foods are not healthy for the body, and even if you choose to eat them, you should only consume them with moderation. Emotional eating, especially indulging in unhealthy food, ends up affecting your weight.

Emotional eating was defined as eating in response to intense emotional emotions. Many studies reveal that having a positive mood can reduce your food intake, so you need to start accepting that positive emotions are now part of emotional eating in the same way that negative emotions are part of it too.

Effects of Emotional Eating

So here are some effects of emotional eating:

Intense Nausea

When you are food binging, the food provides a short-term distraction to the emotions that you are facing, and more than often, you will tend to eat very quickly; as a result, you will overeat. That will then result in stomach pains or nausea, which can last for one or two days. So, it is essential to concentrate on the problem that is causing you stress, instead of eating food to solve that problem.

Feeling Guilty

The next one is feeling guilty. Occasionally, you may use food as a reward to celebrate something that is not necessarily bad. It is essential to celebrate the little wings that you have in life, and if food is the way you choose to celebrate it, you should want to eat healthy meals instead of going for unhealthy meals. However, when food becomes your primary mechanism for coping with emotional stress whenever you feel stressed, upset, lonely, angry, or exhausted, then you will open the fridge and find yourself in an unhealthy cycle, without even being able to target to the root cause of the problem that is making you stressed.

Furthermore, you will be filled with guilt. Even after all the emotional damage has passed away, you will still be filled with remorse for what you have done and the unhealthy lifestyle you choose to make at that moment, which will lower your self-esteem. And then, you will go into another emotional eating outburst.

Weight-Related Health Issues

The next one is weight-related health issues. I'm sure that you are aware of how unhealthy eating affects your weight. Many researchers have discovered that emotional eating affects the weight both positively and negatively. Generally, the foods you crave during those emotional moments are high in sugar, high in salt, and saturated fats. And in those emotional moments, you tend to eat anything that you can lay your hands.

Even though some healthy fast foods are available out there, many are still filled with salt, sugar, and trans-fat content. High carbohydrate food increases the demand for insulin in the body, which then promotes hunger more and more, and therefore you tend to eat more calories than you are supposed to consume. Consuming a high level of fat can have an immediate impact on your blood vessels, and it does that in the short-term. If you consume too much fat, your blood pressure will increase, and you will become hospitable to heart attacks, kidney disease, and another cardiovascular disease. Many manufactured fats are created during food processing, and those fats are found in pizza, dough, crackers, fried pies, cookies, and pastries.

Do not be misinformed; no amount of saturated fat is healthy. If you continue to eat this kind of food, you'll be putting yourself in the risks of HDL and LDL, which is the right kind of cholesterol and the wrong kind of cholesterol. And to be frank, both of them will put your heart into the risk of diabetes, high blood pressure, high cholesterol, obesity, and insulin resistance.

How to Stop Emotional Eating Using Meditation

You already know what to eat, and you already know what not to eat. You already know what is right for your body and what is not suitable for your body. If you're not a nutritionist or a health coach or a fitness activist, you already know these things. When you are alone, you tend to engage in emotional eating, and you successfully keep it to yourself and make sure that no one knows about it. It is just like you surrender your control for food to a food demon, and when that demon possesses you, you become angry, sad, and stressed at once, before you know what is happening, you have gone to your fridge, opened it, and begin to consume whatever is there.

As strong as you, once this food demon has possessed you, it will convince you that food is the only way to get out of that emotional turmoil that you are facing. So, before you know what is happening, you are invading your refrigerator and consuming that jar of almond butter that you promised yourself not to consume. And just a few seconds that you open the jar of almond butter, you take the bottle, put it in your mouth, and close the door again. You do it again and again and again, and before you know what is happening, you have leveled the jar up to halfway, and not a dent has been made on the initial in motion that you were eating over.

Now before you know it, if your consciousness catches up with you. You start to feel sad, guilty, and ashamed. The almond butter that you were eating didn't help you that much, not in the way that you wanted it to help you. So, if there is anything you need to realize, you now feel worse than you were one hour ago. And then, you make a promise that you won't repeat this again and that this is the last time that this will happen.

You promised yourself never to share an entrance with that almond butter again, but then you realize that this is what you have been doing to the gluten-free cookies, to that ice cream, and hot chocolate before now. If this is your behavior, then you'll be able to relate to this. Emotional eating is a healthy addition that you must stop. It is more of a habit and one not easy to control. So, there is hope for you if you are engaging in emotional eating today. You have to be able to have control by yourself and over your emotional eating. There are many strategies that you can use to combat that emotional eating, and one is meditation.

Now when it comes to emotional eating and weight management, it is essential to acknowledge the connection between our minds and our bodies. Today we live in a hectic and packed world that is weighing us down. However, mindful meditation can be a powerful tool to help you to be able to create a rational relationship with the food that you eat. One of the essential things about overcoming emotional eating is not to avoid the emotions, but rather to face them head-on, accept them the way they are and agree that they are a crucial part of your life.

Want to stop emotional eating? Then you need to be able to shift your beliefs and worthiness. You need to be able to create a means to cope with unhealthy situations. It is essential to note that meditation will not cure your emotional eating completely. Instead, it will help you to examine and rationalize all the underlining sensations that are leading to emotional eating in your life. For emotional eaters, the feeling of guilt, shame, and low self-esteem are widespread.

Frequently these negatives create judgment in their mind and trigger unhealthy eating patterns, and they end up feeling like an endless self-perpetuating loop. Meditation helps you to be able to develop a non-judgmental mindset about observing your reality. And that mindset will help you and suppress your emotions negative feelings, without even trying to suppress them or comfort them with foods.

Develop the Mind and Body Connection

Meditation will help you to develop the mind and body connection. And once you're able to create that connection, you will be able to distinguish between emotional eating and physical hunger. Once you can differentiate between that, you'll recognize your cues for hunger and safety. You will instantly tell when your desire is not related to physical hunger. Research indicates that medication will help to strengthen your prefrontal cortex, which is the part of the brain that helps you with will power. That part of the brain is the part of the brain that allows us to resist the urge that is within us. Mindfulness will help the urges to eat even when they're not hungry.

By strengthening that prefrontal cortex, you'll be able to get comfortable at observing those impulses without acting on them. Getting rid of an unhealthy habit and start building new ones, you need to be able to work on your prefrontal cortex, and you can only do that with meditation. Once you start meditating, you will begin reaping the benefits. You will learn how to be able to live more in the present. You'll become more aware of your thinking patterns, and in no time, you will be able to become conscious of how you treat food. You'll be able to make the right choice when it comes to food.

CHAPTER 6:

Affirmation for Healthy Diet and Body Image

Affirmation has to be appreciated, and people should believe in them so that they can work well.

However, for this to work well, you must have a strong belief. Your belief will make you comprehend affirmation for a healthy diet.

You can genuinely achieve all affirmations if, at all, you put more effort and faith in managing. Nothing can't be grasped either conceived, and that's why for you to come up with the best affirmation, then a little effort and faith has to be employed. Before you move further with all these, it would be better for you to understand the real functions or rather the real purpose of affirmation. That's what they do in your daily life. It also appears as their primary function and purpose. The statement will highly motivate you and adds you with more power of urge to move ahead. In this, they not only keep you focused on your daily goals but also maintain that positive feeling in you. In that, they can affect your subconscious and conscious mind. Affirmation always has that hidden ability to change your way of thinking and behaving. That's, they can control or have an effect on how you reason, especially about yourself. As a result of this, you are placing in a better position in which you will be able to transform every part of your world, that's both external and inner worlds. In short, affirmation is all about being extremely positive about yourself and having no space of negative thoughts in your life. You can also define it as having positive and straightforward thinking about yourself. You can also talk of it as an essential phrase that helps you in achieving some of your roles.

Affirmations are always honest words and phrases that you take your little time to speak to yourself. These phrases usually capture your physical health level. Everything that you want in life and how you will achieve them revolves around affirmation. Now that you have known this, you should understand all the statements for a healthy diet and body image in detail form. The following declarations have been approved as the most influential and have been grouped into different categories to help you transparently understand them.

Preparing Meals Affirmation

These affirmations are positive phrases you say to yourself while preparing food. They include the following:

Healthy meal planning is a kind of joy. You derive pleasure in making food that has got everything needed in terms of quality. You feel delighted having prepared all these plans, and this will reflect on how you feel about yourself. The right diet that you planned will boost your morale and gives you that anxious feeling about your body. It implies that planning healthy food or somewhat having a healthy diet plan will help you to have the right ingredients for a better meal.

Many studies have found that the proper meal has a positive effect on your body image in that it improves it to a certain level.

"Hi kitchen, forever my center of nourishment." You look at your kitchen as a center of pleasure where you get all forms of nourishment. When you have positive affirmation thoughts like these, you understand that feeling of relaxed. Do this every day by reassuring yourself that, indeed, your kitchen is just a darling to you. That is the only place where you can get that kind of nourishment your body needed. After that, spend as much as possible time in your darling kitchen. And make yourself a healthy diet that will help you improve not only to your inner world but also to the rest of the external world.

Appreciate your healthy diet. Your diet has helped you a lot in making sure that you can prepare those delicious meals. These meals are not only sumptuous but also highly nutritious. Without your healthy diet, then you couldn't have been in a position to prepare food with such qualities. It is better to note that preparing these kinds of food makes you even healthier. Also, this will make you feel even more joyous, relaxed, and at the end of the day, give you that kind of body shape you have always admired. Remember, healthy diet preparation is the cornerstone of your health. Without this, then you are doomed. Appreciate this affirmation and make it your daily phrase.

A healthy diet enables you to have a healthy meal plan. These meal plans have every ingredient required in making healthy food. You will be in an excellent position to choose from the available options. Having decided, you can now prepare that healthy diet. It will be of great help not only to your body but also to the rest of your environs. It will make you feel kind and more so grateful since the vast diet is at your disposal. It's now you to make a choice, and this will give you peace of mind while choosing. All these will get reflected in your body image. Many authors have tried their best to find why people are always grateful here. Many have failed, while others have concluded that there is that kind of pleasure someone derives from having a wide variety of healthy diets to choose on. Remember, these healthy diets that you have eventually chosen will support your healthy life.

Making nutritious and delicious meals are unavoidable. With a healthy diet within your disposal, you can now affirm yourself that you are in a position to make delicious meals. Meals like these are not only delicious but also are critical requirements in building up your body. Prepare them as many times as you can so that you can realize that shape.

You love having more time in your kitchen. Owning a kitchen for yourself is the first step in realizing your body image. Being in a position to have a healthy diet meal plan comes immediately after the latter. In this situation, you are only required to spend some adorable time in your kitchen just preparing that healthy diet. Affirm yourself that you can manage this behavior, putting more effort into it. Time spent on this has not gone to waste as it helps you make healthy meals. The purpose of these meals has many illustrations and explanations in detail. Having that right healthy diet will require lots of your time. This time you will spend it in your kitchen. Make sure that you make this affirmation your day to day routine and practice it correctly.

Feel the worthiness of your time and money spent on your health. Many people invest in their lives. The main objective here is to help improve their health. You are also supposed to do the same. Invest much in your life, and you should feel that worthiness of every input you plant in your life. Look at the money you have been investing in that health sector and make comparisons with the first time you were not affirming yourself. Is there any change? If yes, then you are worth it; that your money hasn't been wasted or gone into waste. Check on time, especially the one you have invested in your life. How does the body react towards that kind of change? If everything has been positive ever since you started investing, then have an assurance that you have clicked on it, and you are worth it. Your spiritual body and external world should reflect the healthy diet that has been for so long. An improvement will add more value and worthiness to everything. Therefore, this affirmation will help you to improve so much that within a short time, your changes will realize. For you to master this, you can take it as a hobby and recite it every time that you are free, then follow your heart.

You are being in a position to have a choice in anything for the family. In all the aspects of life, from west to east, south to north, your family will come first. Having that basketful of a healthy diet, you will be in the right position to choose all kinds of healthy nutrition for your family.

Healthy food should be part of your family. You should be in a clear position to choose healthy food for you and your family. Your family is part and parcel of your life, and providing them with excellent healthy food will be a blessing. Healthy eating leads to a relaxed mind. You should also note that this will always result in improved body image.

Your kids always appreciate new foods. Try having a change in your diet by providing a new diet. Kids still love different diets, and this will help them to improve on their body image. Eating healthy and making sure that everything is well-prepared initiate the morale of eating, a steering wheel towards your achievements of body image. Remember, it is good to note that healthy new meals motivate you and give you the pleasure of preparing.

Learning new things will make you heal your body. You should struggle as hard as possible to learn new kinds of stuff. New ideas might include modern diets, new cooking styles, and so on. Many studies have concluded that new things will always radiate your body. Your body will glow, and at the end of the day, you will be able to realize a good impression and improvement. Your goals will become a lesser issue since achieving them will be much easier. Your body will also feel some sort of relaxation as the process of healing continues. You will be in a position to feel juvenile, and happiness will be part of your day.

You should have the will to nurture yourself. This phrase will help you manage all the processes leading to nurturing yourself. Never lose hope in this process since it might be tedious. Concentrate on every detail that leads to the nurturing of your body image. After realizing this goal, try as hard as possible to get to bigger goals, which include shedding off more pounds of your weight. The will of nurturing will act as a driving force in your process of preparing healthy meals. According to studies carried out some years back, the intention to nurture yourself is more urging to an extent someone would wish to accomplish it first. However, for you to achieve this, then you need to play a little bit with your kitchen. Your kitchen will give you that kind of motivation and maximum pleasure to prepare that meal.

Eating Meals Affirmation

You need to note down that eating meals affirmations are phrases of great motivation that you tell yourself when you have already made the food. You speak these words always while you are just about to eat. The following statements are forming the eating meals affirmation, which you usually use day in day out.

You must appreciate the food. You have already prepared a delicious meal that you are just about to start eating. Before anything, you need to be grateful for having made such a meal. Appreciating your food will increase that urge even to eat more and cook more. It is also resulting in a kind of motivation that will help you in your daily life. Eating healthy food will make you realize some goals.

CHAPTER 7:

Practicing Hypnosis

We all want time just to relax, dream, and pretend. That refreshes the human body and rejuvenates the soul. It gives us precisely that as we perform our hypnosis: a very intimate moment to enliven and enrich our mind and body. The procedure is over. You need nothing more than a secure and convenient venue.

A Few Simple Rules

There are specific guidelines for hypnosis, and they make sure the method is the most effective and has the most significant advantages. Choose a nice and quiet spot in your home or office when you're about to continue using the recording, where you can relax in a chair, recline or even lay down. Make sure you're comfortable, so you don't have to pay attention to anything else in a spot. Should not listen to your trancework when driving a vehicle or working machinery of some kind, it is essential to agree on a daily period each day or night. Bedtime is a perfect chance to enjoy the trancework, and it can be a fantastic way to get into a restful sleep at this time of the train.

Distractions are possible, and interruptions, instead of making them bother you and pull you off your trancework, using them. To improve the sense of trance, using the sounds of the world around you. E.g., you can hear a noise while doing your hypnosis, and start thinking that this sound distracts you. You then concentrate more on that diversion than on the hypnosis. You may be tempted to combat it—which takes energy off the hypnosis. Instead, when you hear a sound that is disturbing or irritating at first, take control of it by giving it your permission as a background sound to be here. Give it an assignment, such as thinking that "the barking dog's sound helps me go deeper and deeper inside" or "the fan motor sounds like a waterfall that's a soothing background sound." In our private practice in Tucson, there's a day school that inevitably lets the kids play during one of our hypnosis sessions. That is when we say, "Children's music can be a background sound that helps you to go deeper and deeper into yourself now." That is part of our philosophy of "using all."

Distractions also include the sensations you may experience in yourself. You may find yourself feeling, for example, a part of your body that itches. The more you focus on itching or rubbing the itch, the less you concentrate on the trance. You are merely reminding yourself at those moments that you have permission to move your attention back to your trance or daydream and let the itch dissolve. When working with patients with pain disorders, we show them a similar way of focusing attention away from the "distraction" of pain. We can't control the world around us, after all, or the emotions inside of us; however, we can choose where to focus our attention. If you have trouble letting go of an annoying distraction, you may need to order it to be there as a background sound or vibration, helping you to go inside more easily. Detach yourself from anything your commitment to your hypnosis is interfering with. Let go of some dispute with the world. Only let it be there so you won't see it again sooner or later. When you learn to accept a sensation, noise, or another element that interferes with your hypnosis, you don't let it control you any longer.

Law of Reversed Effect

There is a law of hypnosis, called the Reversed Effect Principle, which states that the more you often attempt to do something, the more it doesn't happen. An example is when you want to tell a name that you think you know—it could be a title of a book, a person, a movie—but at the moment you can't say it, and the harder you set goals, the less it is there. The name comes as you say, "I will know later" or "It will come to me later," to your subconscious mind. When letting go of the question, "What is the word? What name is it?" You activated your subconscious mind to get the answer right now, and it always does. So, the Reversed Effect Rule is that it only gives you the opposite (the reverse) when you are trying too hard for something.

Simple Techniques

Getting lost in your thoughts and ideas is that a soft trip into the core of yourself is called "going into a trance." Basic self-hypnosis methods involve going into a trance, deepening the trance, using that trance state to give mental-body signals and feedback, and coming out of the trance.

Entering Trance

I will be your mentor when you use the trancework on the audio as you go into a trance. I'll use a form of trance induction that you will find relaxing and concentrating. You undoubtedly saw the spinning watch technique on television, which I have never seen anybody use in thirty-five years of experience. Still, there are many different ways to concentrate your mind on slipping into a trance. You can look at a wall spot, use a breathing technique, or use the gradual relaxation of the body.

On the audio trancework, you'll hear a range of induction methods. These are simply the signs or signals you send yourself to say, "I'm going into a trance" or "I'm going to do my hypnosis now." Going into a trance can also be thought of as "making yourself daydream... intentionally."

You're letting yourself be immersed in your thoughts and ideas, really distracted, and encouraging yourself to think or visualize what you want to do and what you want to accomplish. There is no "going under." Instead, there is a beautiful experience of going inside.

Deepening the Trance

Deepening your trance lets you digest your thoughts, ideas, and learn more. That is done with progressive relaxation: going "deeper and deeper inside..." with images or scenes, for example, or counting a sequence of numbers. We want to propose that you create a vertical picture synonymous with moving lower, such as a path leading down a mountain or into a lush green gorge, when you hear the counting from 10 down to 0. You can visualize or envision going further into a scene or location that's much more fun and relaxing for you when you hear me count. We say this with "deepening the trance."

Talking to the Mind of Your Body with Messages and Suggestions

You'll hear my voice speaking two areas of your mind during the trancework. Your conscious thought mind is a part of the soul. That's the part of you that's great at telling time, making change, learning how to read and write; it's the "conscious mind." The thinking mind will continue to do its regular activity of having thoughts throughout the trancework. Right now, you don't have to worry about cleaning your head, or emptying your head, or fully setting your mind in order. Only note that your mind begins to "dream," and your task is only to unplug or disconnect entirely that you don't have to respond to those feelings. You owe them permission to continue streaming. For example, if your "to do" list keeps coming up, just let it float past, instead of focusing on it. The other part of your mind that I'm trying to refer to is what we call your subconscious mind—"sub" as it's below your awareness level of thought. Your subconscious mind can control the trillions of cells in your body, your body chemistry, and all of the body's metabolism, digestion, nervous system, endocrine system, and immune system functions. The mind-body has a tremendous amount of experience, and you gain and acquire additional knowledge in doing the hypnosis so your body's mind can function upon, aligned with your inspiration, beliefs, and expectations, to support you with your weight loss.

You also can adapt and customize the words that are spoken or the pictures that are portrayed to suit you best. The cycle of tailoring is critical. Because it is the self-hypnosis, it must suit you, and all hypnosis is self-hypnosis. Hypnosis, as we have said, is not something that you do. It is something you are being guided to experience, and you are learning it as you experience it. Repetition and training build in your strong ability and knowledge. You can also term it subconscious awareness, as your subconscious mind will do it for you without you having to think about it. So the thoughts and ideas that might have troubled you about your weight, or your weight loss inability, are now being changed into something that supports your perfect body. And the mind-body memorizes, so that rather than the unwelcome effects of the past, it may return to the mind.

For starters, if you believe you're a "yo-yo" dietitian, if you've still recovered the weight you've lost, you can use your trancework to say, "I lose weight every day, and my body knows how to make this a lasting capacity. I'm enjoying my ideal weight." Subconscious awareness, or mind-body experience gained from your trancework, is just like learning to ride a bike or drive a car. As you first heard, there appeared to be a lot of things to pay attention to at the same time, but your mind-body soon focused on this information, and you can drive confidently today, so you don't even have to remind your feet what to do.

CHAPTER 8:

Mind Meditation

The Joyful Mind Meditation

This meditation can be used for a time of stress and anxiety. It will help guide you into a more relaxed state where you can focus on the present and find inner peace. Please use this meditation method when you find your mind racing. That can also be used if you feel like you are about to have an anxiety or panic attack.

"Welcome to the joyful mind guided meditation.

Please find yourself in a quiet area to sit and dim the lighting.

Make sure you are comfortable. Just sit your back straight and relaxed. Loosen any tight clothing that may be restricting you.

Let your hands lie loosely and relaxed into your lap. Close your eyes and take a deep breath. Now, relax.

Now that your eyes are closed, you may begin to connect with your inner self of thoughts and feelings.

Gradually, let the outside world fade from your awareness.

For the next few minutes, allow yourself to enjoy and submerge into this relaxing experience.

You are free from all your responsibilities during this meditation. Any thoughts, tasks, or concerns that you may have do not require your immediate attention. Tuck those thoughts away and focus on your inner thoughts.

You may find that your mind will begin to wander during this meditation. That is okay, and this is normal. Just bring your awareness back to the present and the sound of my voice. These will guide you into a place of inner peace and deep relaxation.

Remember that you are in charge of yourself. If you wish to end this meditation, you can do so by opening your eyes.

Begin to take a slow, long, and deep breath in through your nose. Release that breath through your mouth.

Find your inner self begin to relax.

Begin to take another deep breath in, and exhale.

Notice how calm this type of breathing is. Be aware of the feelings of relaxation starting to spread throughout your body. Starting from your lungs, all the way down to your toes.

Continue to breathe deeply, slowly, and gently. Try not to breathe too quickly.

With each inhale and exhale, your thoughts start to become lighter.

Now, you start to feel a sense of spaciousness inside of you. It will open up slowly.

Keep relaxing.

Let the soft movement of your breath to guide you into an even more relaxed state of being.

Breathe in. Breathe out. Deeper you go into this state of relaxation.

Breathe in. Breathe out. Let your mind gradually slow down. Breathe in. Breathe out. Let it slow down some more.

Breathe in. Breathe out.

You may now begin to enjoy a guided journey into your inner place of joy and serenity.

Allow images and visualizations to form in your mind naturally, as I speak. Do so at your own pace.

Begin to let your expectations drift away from you. Let them go. Allow yourself to experience this meditation journey in whatever form comes naturally to you.

Begin to imagine that you are standing in a green and beautiful grassy field. The field stretches on for miles. You can feel the heat of the sun on your face, slowly warming your body.

You feel the soft and lush green grass, cushioning your bare feet. Right now, you can smell the nature all around you.

You can hear the sounds of nature around you, the rustling of the blowing grass. Birds were singing—the rustling of leaves in the distance.

You feel very much at home in this serene place.

You have the time in the world.

You're safe and happy here.

Take a moment to appreciate your surroundings.

You notice a sizeable luscious tree growing close by.

You begin to walk towards that tree.

Take your time walking. There is no rush whatsoever. Stay in the moment and appreciate the feeling of each step.

As you walk towards the tree, you feel yourself falling more deeply into a state of relaxation.

You are now standing under the tree. It's long branches, and large leaves hang right above your head.

You notice that the tree holds many delicious fruits in all shapes, sizes, and colors.

That is not just an ordinary tree. Its fruits carry special powers.

Reach your arm up and take a piece of fruit from the branches. Watch it for a moment. Notice the color of this fruit, the texture, and the weight. It's quite heavy in your hand.

Take a bite of this fruit.

As you swallow the fruit, it slides down your throat and into your belly. You begin to feel something beautiful happen.

A feeling of happiness and peace begins to glow inside of your body.

The sensation starts in your abdomen, and it spreads to your chest and into your heart.

Let go of thinking, and begin to bring all your attention on feeling. Embellish in the sensation of joy, love, and peace. Feel your body gently glowing with these feelings.

Take another bite of the magical fruit, taste it.

This wonderful feeling begins to intensify even more.

Feel yourself begin to radiate this wonderful sensation to love and happiness.

Take another bite of the fruit. Take as many bites as you'd like.

Relax and let yourself drown in this enchanting feeling. Instead of trying, just let it effortlessly take over. Break down any walls that you feel comfortable breaking and let it surround you as much as you like.

Stay with these joyful and peaceful feelings. Enjoy this time of meditation.

You may remain in this relaxed state of meditation for as long as you please. Don't feel rushed to leave."

When you are ready, you may finish this meditation. Simple open your eyes to leave. Take a deep breath and give yourself a few moments to adjust before standing up.

The Spiritual Meditation

This meditation is used for those who want to explore spirituality further. You may not feel any different during this meditation, but you will feel the physical and mental benefits of this practice. During this meditation, you will have to be awake. This technique can lead to sleep. Avoid that to experience spiritual effects.

Before we begin this meditation, think about your spirituality. What gives you meaning in life? You will need to conceptualize a word or a short phrase that gives you meaning. You will repeat those words during the time it takes to exhale a breath. For example, if nature holds deep and strong meaning for you, you may select phrases that relate to it.

"Welcome to spiritual meditation.

Find a comfortable position for you, one that allows you to remain awake.

Let's begin.

Close your eyes. Choose to focus your gaze on a small area. Start by relaxing your muscles and relieving any tension you feel.

When you feel thoughts come to your mind, simply acknowledge them and let it pass. Bring your attention back to your body.

Bring your awareness to your breathing. Notice the way each breath feels; let it be natural. Just observe.

As thoughts arise in your mind, acknowledge them and let it go. Return your attention to breathing.

Breathe slowly, deeply, and naturally.

If you find your thoughts wandering some more, bring your attention to breathing.

Notice how your breath flows gently in and out through your body. It feels effortless.

Interruptions are normal. You may find yourself thinking about other thoughts. Let them go, and focus on breathing.

Now, begin to think about the meaningful words or phrases you've selected. Begin to say this word in your mind as you breathe out.

Each time you exhale, repeat the phrase.

Continue repeating the phrase every time you breathe out.

With each breath, allow distracting thoughts to float by your awareness.

Let any spiritual feeling linger in your body. Don't ignore it, but let it brew deeply inside you. Let is consume your body and let it stay.

Repeat the phrase. Feel the spirituality within you intensify. You may leave this meditation at any moment, simply open your eyes.

Let your body communicate and get comfortable with the feeling of spirituality.

Breathe in. Breathe out. Let your thoughts turn to your body. You were relaxed, peaceful, and calm. Notice how your body feels as it becomes more aware of your surroundings.

Bring your attention back to your thoughts. Bring it back to your regular conscious awareness. You may let the spirituality leave your body.

Stay seated for a few more moments with your eyes open. Enjoy the feeling of reawakening. Savor the relaxation and all the other emotions you've encountered.

Begin to reflect on the experience of spiritual meditation. Be aware of all the feelings during the practice. You should be feeling free from worries.

End this guided meditation by wiggling your toes and then your fingers. Stretch your back and shoulders. When you are ready, you may stand up and continue with your day."

The Gratitude Meditation

The gratitude meditation is used as a conscious effort to appreciate all the things in the world that makes us feel good. It is directly related to opening our hearts and embracing all our blessings. This meditation is very popular amongst Buddhist monks and nuns. It's typically practiced at the beginning and end of their days to pay gratitude to everything that helped them throughout that day, and this also includes their sufferings.

Gratitude meditation gives us the power we need to face our problems and weaknesses to acknowledge the darker parts of life. This meditation can be used when you are feeling the burdens of the world. Try this guided meditation when you feel self-pity or hopelessness.

Before you begin this meditation, think about something in your life that you are grateful for; think about where that feeling is held in your body. You can feel thankful for your home, spouse, or even the vacation you just purchased.

"Welcome to the gratitude meditation.

Find a comfortable sitting position and dim the lighting.

I will begin by bringing your awareness to the things you are grateful for in life.

Give the sense of gratitude the chance to come up naturally. When it arises, let yourself sink into that feeling. Surrender yourself to it. Begin to notice how it feels inside your body, how that energy feels. If the feeling of gratitude does not come up immediately, don't try to force yourself, it is okay. Instead, just surrender yourself to your heart and not your head."

CHAPTER 9:

Hypnosis Script

A t this point in the audio, I invite you to make yourself as comfortable as possible in your bed. Please have all the light's turned off and distractions put away. You have already set in a full, hard day of work. Think of sleeping sound and comfortable through the night as a reward for working so hard.

- How was your day today?

- Were you productive?

- How did you feel?

Gently tuck yourself under the cover, and we will begin our journey. Ready?

Inhale deeply. Hold onto that breath for a moment, and then let it go. To begin, I am going to lead you through an induction script for self-hypnosis. By allowing yourself to slip into this state of mind, it will help you just let go of your stress that your holding to, even if it is in your subconscious. I am going to help you tap into these emotions so you can let them go and sleep like you never have before.

All of us are stressed. Honestly, who can sleep when worried? In this state of mind, you probably feel too alert to even think about sleeping. When you are stressed, the adrenal glands in your body release adrenaline and cortisol. Both of these hormones keep you awake and stop you from falling asleep.

In the audio to follow, we will go over letting go of your worries, even if it is just for the night. You are in a safe place right now. Anything you need to get done can wait until tomorrow. You must take this time for yourself. We need a break from reality at some point or another. I invite you now to take another deep breath so we can focus on what is crucial right now; sleep.

To start, I would like you to close your eyes gently, as you do this, wiggle slightly until your body feels comfortable in your bed. When you find your most comfortable position, it is time to begin breathing.

While you're focusing on your breath, remind yourself to breathe slow and deep. Feel as the air fills your lungs and release it comfortably. Feel as your body relaxes further under the sheets. You begin to feel a warm glow, wrapping your whole body in a comfortable blanket.

Before you let go into a deep hypnotic state, listen carefully to the words I am saying at this moment.

Everything is going to happen automatically.

At this moment, there is nothing you need to focus on; you will have no control over what happens next in our session. But you are okay with that. At this moment, you are warm and safe. You are preparing your body for a full night's rest and letting go of any thoughts you may have future or the past. What matters the most is your comfort, your breath, and the incredible sleep you are about to experience.

Now, feel as the muscles around your eyes begin to relax. I invite you to continue breathing deeply and bring your attention to your eyes. They are beginning to feel heavy and relaxed. Your eyes worked hard for you today. They watched as you worked, they kept you safe as you walked around, and they showed other people you were paying attention to them as you spoke. Thank your eyes at this moment and allow them to rest for the night so they will be prepared for tomorrow.

Your breath is coming easy and free now. Soon, you will enter a hypnotic trance with no effort. This trance will be deep, peaceful, and safe. There is nothing for your conscious mind to do at this moment. Allow for your subconscious mind to take over and do the work for you. This trance will come automatically. Soon, you will feel like you are dreaming. Allow yourself to relax and give in to my voice. All you need to focus on is my voice. You are doing wonderfully. Without noticing, you have already changed your rate of breath. You are breathing easy and free. There is no thought involved. Your body knows what you need to do, and you can relax further into your subconscious mind.

Now, you are starting to show signs of drifting off into this peaceful hypnotic trance. I invite you to enjoy the sensations as your subconscious mind takes over and listens to the words I am speaking to you. It is slowly becoming less important for you to listen to me. Your subconscious listens, even as I begin to whisper.

You are drifting further and further away. You are becoming more relaxed and more comfortable. At this moment, nothing is bothering you. Your inner mind is listening to me, and you are beginning to realize that you don't care about slipping into a deep trance.

This peaceful state allows you to be comfortable and relaxed. Being hypnotized is pleasant and enjoyable. That is beginning to feel natural for you. Each time I hypnotize you, it becomes more enjoyable than the time before.

You will enjoy these sensations; you are comfortable, peaceful. You are entirely calm.

As we progress through the relaxing exercises, you will learn something new about yourself. You are working gently to develop your sleep techniques without even knowing you are developing them in the first place.

Slip completely into your mental state. When I say number three, your brain is going to take over, and you will find yourself in the forest. This forest is peaceful, calm, and serene. It is safe and comfortable, much like your bed at this moment.

As you inhale, try to bring more oxygen into your body with beautiful, deep breaths. As you exhale, feel as your body relaxes more and more into the bed. Breathing comes easy and free for you. Like you, you are becoming more peaceful and calmer without even realizing it.

As we continue, you do not care how relaxed you are. You are happy in the state of mind. You do not have a care in the world. Your subconscious mind is always aware of the words I am saying to you. As we go along, it is becoming less important for you to listen to my voice.

Your inner mind is receiving everything I tell you. Your conscious mind is relaxed and peaceful. As you find your peace of mind, we will begin to explore this forest you have found yourself in, together.

Imagine lying near a stream in this beautiful and peaceful forest. It is a sunny, warm summer day. As you lay comfortably in the grass beside this stream, you feel a warm breeze gently moving through your hair. Inhale deep and experience how fresh and clean this air is. Inhale again and exhale. Listen carefully as the stream flows beside you. A quiet whoosh noise, filling your ears and relaxing you even further. Listen to me. Your subconscious mind takes hold and listens to everything I am saying. Enjoy the beautiful nature around you. The sunlight shines through the trees and kisses your skin gently. The birds begin to sing a happy tune. You smile, feeling yourself become one with nature.

Each time you exhale, I want to imagine your whole body relaxing more. You are becoming more at ease. As you do this, I want you to begin to use your imagination. You are lying on the grass. It is located in a green meadow with the sun shining down on you. The sun is not hot, but a comfortable warm.

Imagine that beautiful flowers are blooming everywhere around you. Watch as the flowers move gently in the breeze. Their scents waft toward your nose as you inhale deeply and exhale.

Imagine that you begin to stand up. As you do this, you look over your left shoulder gently, and you see a mountain near the edge of the beautiful meadow, a trip up to the top of the mountain to see this beautiful view from a different angle.

As you begin to walk, you follow the stream. Imagine gently bending over and placing your hand, not the cool, rushing water. As you look upon the sea, imagine how clean and cool this water is. The stream flows gently across your fingers, and it relaxes you.

When you are ready, we will head toward the mountain again. As you grow closer to the mountain, the birds begin to chirp. Inhale deep and imagine how the pine trees smell around you. Soon, you begin to climb the mountain at a comfortable pace.

You are enjoying the trip. It is beautiful to be outside with this beautiful nature, taking in all the sights and sounds. The meadow grows smaller as you climb higher, but you are not afraid. The scene is gorgeous from up here, and you are happy at this moment.

As you reach the top, take a deep breath and pat yourself on the back for your accomplishment. Take a look down on the meadow and see how small the trees look.

The breeze is blowing your hair around gently, and the sun continues to shine down on the top of your head. Imagine that you are taking a seat at the very top of the mountain and take a few moments to appreciate this nature. You wish you could always be this relaxed.

When you take your life into your own hands, you will be able to. That is why we are here. Of course, you may be here because you want to sleep, but you can't do that truly unless you learn how to let go of your stress. Through guided meditation and exercises within this audio, you will learn how to become a better version of yourself.

Soon, we will work on deepening your trance. You are beginning to relax further into the meditation and opening your heart and soul to the practice. Remember that you are safe, and you are happy to be here.

CHAPTER 10:

Script 1 – Self-Hypnosis Relaxation Techniques

George taught Bonnie a hundred useful positive affirmations for weight loss and to keep her motivated. She chose the ones that she wanted to build in her program and used them every day. She was losing weight very slowly, which bothered her very much. She thought she was going in the wrong direction and was about to give up, but George told her not to be worried since its completely natural speed. It takes time for the subconscious to collate all the information and start working according to her conscious will. Also, her body remembered the fast weight loss, but her subconscious remembered her emotional damage, and now it is trying to prevent it. In reality, after some months of hard work, she started to see the desired results. She weighed 74 kilos (163 lbs). According to dietitians, the success of dieting is greatly influenced by how people talk the use of "I should" or "I must" is to be avoided whenever possible. Anyone who says, "I shouldn't eat French fries" or "I have to get a bite of chocolate" will feel that they have no control over the events. Instead, if you say "I prefer" to leave the food, you will feel more power and less guilt. The term "dieting" should be avoided. Proper nutrition should be seen as a permanent lifestyle change. For example, the correct wording is, "I've changed my eating habits" or "I'm eating healthier."

Diets are fattening. Why?

The body needs fat. Our body wants to live, so it stores fat. Removing this amount of fat from the body is not as easy as the body protects against weight loss. During starvation, our bodies switch to a 'saving flame,' burning fewer calories to avoid starving. Those who are starting to lose weight are usually optimistic, as, during the first week, they may experience 1-3 kg (2-7 lbs) of weight loss, which validates their efforts and suffering. However, their body has deceived them very well because it does not want to break down fat. Instead, it begins to break down muscle tissue. At the beginning of dieting, our bodies burn sugar and protein, not fat. Burned sugar removes a lot of water out of the body; that's why we experience amazing results on the scale. It should take about seven days for our body to switch to fat burning. Then our body's alarm bell rings. Most diets have a sad end: reducing your metabolic rate to a lower level. That means that if you only eat a little more afterward, you regain all the weight you have lost previously. After dieting, the body will make special efforts to store fat for the impending famine.

We must understand what our soul needs. Those who desire to have success must first and foremost change their spiritual foundation. It is important to pamper our souls during a period of weight loss. All overweight people tend to rag on themselves for eating forbidden food, "I have overeaten again. My willpower is so weak!"

Imagine a person very close to you who has gone through a difficult time while making mistakes from time to time. Are we going to scold or try to help and motivate them? If we love them, we would instead comfort them and try to convince them to continue. No one tells their best friend that they are weak, ugly, or bad, just because they are struggling with their weight. If you don't say it to someone, don't do so to yourself either! Let us be aware of this: during weight loss, our soul needs peace and support. All bad opinions, even if they are only expressed in thought, are detrimental and divert us from our purpose. You must support yourself with positive reinforcement. There is no place for the all or nothing principle. A single piece of cake will not ruin your entire diet. Realistic thinking is more useful than disaster theory. A cookie is not the end of the world. Eating should not be a reward. Cakes should not make up for a bad day. If you are generally a healthy consumer, eat some goodies sometimes because of its delicious taste and to pamper your soul.

I'll give you a hundred positive affirmations you can use to reinforce your weight loss. I'll divide them into main categories based on the most typical situations for which you need confirmation. You can repeat all of them whenever you need to, but you can choose the ones that are more suitable for your circumstances. If you prefer to listen to them during meditation, you can record them with a piece of beautiful, relaxing music.

General Affirmations to Reinforce Your Well-Being

1. Thank you for making me happy today.

2. Today is a perfect day. I meet friendly and helpful people, whom I treat kindly.

3. Every new day is for me. I live to make myself feel good. Today I just pick good thoughts for myself.

4. Something wonderful is happening to me today.

5. I feel good.

6. I am calm, energetic, and cheerful.

7. My organs are healthy.

8. I am satisfied and balanced.

9. Living in peace and understanding with everyone.

10. I listen to others with patience.

11. In every situation, I find the good.

12. I accept and respect myself and my fellow human beings.

13. I trust myself; I trust my inner wisdom.

Do you often scold yourself? Then repeat the following affirmations frequently:

14. I forgive myself.

15. I'm good to myself.

16. I motivate myself over and over again.

17. I'm doing my job well.

18. I care about myself.

19. I am doing my best.

20. Very proud of myself for my achievements.

21. I am aware that sometimes I have to pamper my soul.

22. I remember that I did a great job this week.

23. I deserved this small piece of candy.

24. I have to let go of the feeling of guilt.

25. I release the blame.

26. Everyone is imperfect. I accept that I am too.

If you feel pain when you choose to avoid delicious food, you need to motivate yourself with affirmations:

27. I am motivated and persistent.

28. I control my life and my weight.

29. I'm ready to change my life.

30. Changes make me feel better.

31. I follow my diet with joy and cheerfulness.

32. I am aware of my amazing capacities.

33. I am grateful for my opportunities.

34. Today I'm excited to start a new diet.

35. I always keep in mind my goals.

36. I imagine myself slim and beautiful.

37. Today I am happy to have the opportunity to do what I have long been postponing.

38. I possess the energy and will to go through my diet.

39. I prefer to lose weight instead of wasting time on momentary pleasures.

Here you can find affirmations that help you to change serious convictions and blockages:

40. I see my progress every day.

41. I listen to my body's messages.

42. I'm taking care of my health.

43. I eat healthy food.

44. I love who I am.

45. I love how life supports me.

46. A good parking space, coffee, conversation. It's all for me today.

47. It feels good to be awake because I can live in peace, health, love.

48. I'm grateful that I woke up. I take a deep breath of peace and tranquillity.

49. I love my body. I love being served by me.

50. I eat by tasting every flavor of the food.

51. Being aware of the benefits of healthy food.

52. I enjoy eating healthy food and being fitter every day.

53. I feel energetic because I eat well.

Many people are struggling with being overweight because they don't move enough. The very root of this issue can be a refusal to do exercises due to negative biases in our minds.

We can overcome these beliefs by repeating the following affirmations:

54. I like moving because it helps my body burn fat.

55. Each time I exercise, I am getting closer to having a beautiful, tight shapely body.

56. It's a very uplifting feeling of being able to climb up to 100 steps without stopping.

57. It's easier to have an excellent quality of life if I move.

58. I like the feeling of returning to my home tired but happy after a long winter walk.

59. Physical exercises help me have a longer life.

60. I am proud to have better fitness and agility.

61. I feel happier thanks to the happiness hormone produced by exercise.

62. I feel full thanks to the enzymes that produce a sense of fullness during physical exercises.

63. I am aware even after exercise, my muscles continue to burn fat, and so I lose weight while resting.

64. I feel more energetic after exercise.

65. My goal is to lose weight. Therefore I exercise.

66. I am motivated to exercise every day.

67. I lose weight while I exercise.

List of generic affirmations that you can build in your program:

68. I'm glad I'm who I am.

69. Today, I read articles and watch movies that make me feel positive about my diet progress.

70. I love it when I'm happy.

71. Taking a deep breath to enhance my fears.

72. Today I do not want to prove my truth, but I want to be happy.

73. I am strong and healthy. I'm fine, and I'm getting better.

74. I am happy today because whatever I do, I find joy in it.

75. I pay attention to what I can become.

76. I love myself and I'm helpful to others.

77. I accept what I cannot change.

78. I am contented that I can eat healthy food.

79. I am happy that I have been changing my life with my new healthy lifestyle.

80. Avoid comparing myself to others.

81. I accept and support who I am and turn to me with love.

82. Today I can do anything for my improvement.

83. I'm fine. I'm happy for life. I love who I am. I'm strong and confident.

84. I am calm and satisfied.

85. Today is perfect for me to exercise and to be healthy.

86. I have decided to lose weight, and I am strong enough to follow my will.

87. I love myself, so I want to lose weight.

88. I am proud of myself because I follow my diet program.

89. I see how much stronger I am.

90. I know that I can do it.

CHAPTER 11:

Script 2 – Strengthen the Experience

How Does It Feel Loving Yourself?

Have a look at these characteristics. Are these familiar to you? It is the way it will feel for those who like yourself:

- You genuinely feel happy and accepting your world, even though you might not agree with everything within it.

- You're compassionate with your flaws or less-than-perfect behaviors, understanding that you're capable of improving and changing.

- You mercifully love compliments and feel joyful inside.

- You frankly see your flaws and softly accept them learning to alter them.

- You accept all of the goodness that comes your way.

- You honor the great qualities and the fantastic qualities of everybody around you.

- You look at the mirror while seeing your face smiling (at least all the period).

Many confound self-love with becoming arrogant and greedy. But some individuals are so caught up in themselves they make the tag of being egotistical and thinking just of these. We do not find that as a healthful indulgent, however, as a character that's not well balanced in enjoying love and loving others. It's not selfish to get things your way; however, it's egotistical to insist that everybody else can see them your way too. The Dalai Lama states, "If you do not enjoy yourself, then you can't love other people. You won't have the capacity to appreciate others. If you don't have any empathy on your own, then you aren't capable of developing empathy for others." Dr. Karl Menninger, a psychologist, states it this way: "Self-love isn't opposed to this love of different men and women. You cannot truly enjoy yourself and get yourself a favor with no people a favor, and vice versa." We're referring to the healthiest type of self-indulgent, that simplifies the solution to accepting your best good.

Have a better look at the way you see your flaws and blame yourself. Self-love and finding an error or depriving yourself aren't in any way compatible. If you suppress or refuse to enjoy yourself, you're in danger of paying too much focus on your flaws, that is a sort of self-loathing. You don't want to place focus on negative aspects of yourself, for holding these ideas in your mind, and you're giving them the psychological energy which brings that result or leaves it actual.

Self-hypnosis can help you use your mind-body to make new and much more loving ideas and beliefs on your own. It helps your mind-body create and take fluctuations in the patterns of feeling and thinking about what has been for you for quite a while, and which aren't helpful for you. The trancework about the sound incorporates many positive suggestions to change your ideas, emotions, and beliefs in alignment with your ideal weight.

An integral goal for all these positive hypnotic suggestions is the innermost feeling of enjoying yourself. In case your self-loving feelings are constant with your ideal weight, then it is going to occur with increased ease. But if you harbor bitterness or remorse, or sense undeserving, these emotions operate contrary to enjoying yourself enough to think and take your ideal weight. Lucille Ball stated it well: "Love yourself first, and everything falls inline."

The hypnotic suggestions about the sound are directions for change that led to the maximum "internal" degree of mind-body or unconscious. However, the "outer" changes in lifestyle activity should also happen. Many weight-loss approaches you have been using might appear to be a lot of work. We suggest that by adopting a mindset that's without the psychological pressure related to "needing to," "bad or good," or even "simple or hard," with no judgment in any way, the fluctuations could be joyous. Yes, joyous. That produces the whole journey of earning adjustments and shifting easier. The term "a labor of love" implies you enjoy doing this so much, and it isn't labor or responsibility. The "labor" of organizing a family feast in a vacation season, volunteering at a hospital or school, or even buying a present for someone exceptional can appear effortless. Here is the mindset that will assist you in following some weight loss procedures. We want you to just place yourself in the situation of being adored. You're doing so to you. Loving yourself eliminates the job, and that means it is possible to relish your advancement toward a lifestyle that encourages your ideal weight. Think about some action that you like to perform. Imagine yourself performing this action today. Notice that when you're doing something which you like to do, you're feeling energized and enjoyable, and some other attempt is evidenced by enjoyment, "loving what you're doing." Sometimes, we recommend that you also find that as "enjoying yourself doing this." Maybe by directing a more favorable attitude toward enjoying yourself, you'll end up enjoying what you're doing.

Lisa's Brimming Smile

After Lisa and Rick wed, both have been slender and appreciated for their active lifestyles, which included softball and Pilates classes at the local gym. When their very first baby was born, Lisa had obtained an additional fifteen lbs. And now, their second baby came three years after, and she was twenty pounds overweight. Depending on the demands of motherhood depended on fast-frozen foods, canned foods, and table food. Persistent sleep deprivation also let her power level reduced, and she can hardly keep up with the toddlers. Rick, a promising young company executive, took more duties on the job, increasing the"ladder of success," indulging in company lunches, and even working late afternoon. He'd return home late, watched the T.V., and eat leftover pizza.

The youthful couple accepted their old way of life but observed with dismay as their bodies grew tired and old beyond their years. However, they lasted. If their oldest boy entered astronomy, they would become more upset. Small Ricky appeared to be the goal of each germfree, and he started to miss several days of college. If this was not enough, he also attracted the germs to the house to his small brother, mother, and father. It appeared that four of these were with them the whole winter.

The infant was colicky. From the spring, following a household bout with influenza, Lisa's friend supplied the title of a behavioral therapist to whom she explained about the ability to shed some light on the recurrent diseases of Lisa's small boys. In the first consultation, Lisa declared the previous four decades of her household's life, culminating at current influenza where the small boys were recuperating. They were exhausted, tired, not sleeping well, and usually under sunlight. With summer vacation just around the corner, Lisa had been distressed to receive her family back on the right track.

The words of the nutritionist were straightforward: Start feeding yourself along with your household foods, which are fresh and ready in your home. Start buying fruits and veggies, and make some simple recipes using rice and other grains. Learn how to create healthy and wholesome dishes for your loved ones. These phrases triggered Lisa to remember when she had been a kid about the time of her very own small boys. She remembered her mother fixing large fruit salads using lemon. She recalled delicious dishes of homemade soup along with hot fresh bread. Instantly, Lisa knew what she needed to do for her boys.

And she'd make it happen. Approximately six months after, we received a telephone call from Lisa. I can hear the grin brimming in her voice. "You cannot think the shift in our loved ones. Ricky has had just one cold in the past six weeks. We are all sleeping much better, and also, the baby is happy and sleeping during the night. Four days per week, we have a family walk after breakfast or after dinner. And guess what? I have lost thirty-five lbs, and I was not dieting! I'm better than I have ever felt."

Giving Forth

Forgiveness is a significant step in enjoying yourself. At any time you forgive, you're "committing forth" or "letting go" of a thing you're holding inside you. Let's be clear about this: bias is simply for you, not anybody else. It's not a kind of accepting, condoning, or justifying somebody else's activities. It's a practice of letting go of an adverse impression that has remained within you too long. It's letting go of any emotion or idea, which can be an obstacle between you and enjoying yourself and getting what you desire.

A lot of us are considerably more crucial and harder on ourselves than we're about others. When you continue with the notions of what you need or shouldn't have completed, you aren't enjoying yourself. Instead, you're putting alert energy to negative beliefs about yourself. Ideas like "I must have taken a stroll" or even "I should not have eaten this second slice of pie" can also be regarded as self-punishing. Sometimes, penalizing yourself, either by lack of overeating or eating, may even lead to a discount for your well-being. By changing your focus to self-appreciation, you go from the negative to the positive, which is quite a bit more conducive to self-loving.

Writing a diary about all choices you make every day may promote self-improvement. By forgiving yourself and forgiving other people, you launch the psychological hold that previous events might have had to you personally, and you also make yourself accessible to appreciate yourself. When you launch the effects of previous encounters by forgiving, then you undergo reassurance and a calm comfort on your body, which helps you take your ideal weight.

Basic Rules of Self – Hypnosis Diet

- No explanations

- No denying

- No criticizing

Negative thoughts, thoughts, and expressions aren't permitted on your understanding (or maybe not for long, anyhow). Remember, there are no mistakes, just lessons. Love yourself, hope on your options, and what's possible.

CHAPTER 12:

Script 3 – How to Use Guided Meditation and Positive Affirmations for Weight Loss

Have you attempted and neglected to get in shape? In this case, you realize how troublesome it very well may be to stay with a weight loss program. What's more, in any event, when you do figure out how to drop those additional pounds, keeping them off is another fight together. In any case, you don't need to spend a mind-blowing remainder doing combating with your willpower with an end goal to get and stay thin.

One of the critical contrasts between those individuals who figure out how to get more fit and keep it off effectively, and the individuals who don't, is that the previous gathering changes their eating and exercises propensities as well as their mindset too.

If your mind isn't your ally, getting more fit will be troublesome or inconceivable because you'll be continually undermining your endeavors. How about we investigate required for the sort of mindset that prompts lasting, sound weight loss?

Persistence

Right off the bat, you should show restraint. The individuals who shed pounds gradually and consistently are well on the way to keep it off. So overlook each one of those diet designs that guarantee you can drop 10 pounds or more in seven days—the vast majority of that will be water weight, and will recover right when you begin eating ordinarily. It's just human to need a convenient solution; however, if you need to lose the weight, keep it off and move on without having to battle with your body for an incredible remainder continually, it merits adopting the moderate strategy, since compromising makes weight loss increasingly troublesome and tedious over the long haul.

Adaptability

Adaptability is likewise significant for effective long haul weight loss. If you make amazingly rigid guidelines about what you can and can't eat, you may get more fit, yet risks are that you'll be hopeless. You're probably not going to adhere to those principles for an incredible remainder. What's more, when you have this 'win or bust' sort of mindset, and you disrupt your guidelines even somewhat, it very well may be enticing to go on a hard and fast binge a short time later, because all things considered, you've blitz now! Then again, if you follow reasonable rules while recognizing that there will be times (for example, occasions and unique events) when you'll eat food that isn't a piece of your ordinary diet. At that point, these 'illegal nourishments' will appear to be less appealing because they're not something that you've restricted from your life forever.

Consistency

Consistency is another piece of a fruitful weight loss mindset. That may appear to repudiate the above point. However, it doesn't generally. Interestingly, you eat heartily and follow your activity plan most of the time. Along these lines, you'll stay away from yo-yo and unfortunate practices, for example, the binge/starve cycle. It's the moves you make most of the time that will give you the outcomes you are looking on. When you're focused on building long haul changes in your way of life, instead of searching for a convenient solution, you'll increasingly spur to embrace a moderate and adjusted arrangement that you can try reliably.

Self-Love

It is additionally imperative to have an inspirational mentality towards yourself. Presently in case you're similar to a great many people who need to shed pounds, odds are you don't feel generally excellent about your body and appearance. While you don't need to claim to cherish something that you loathe about yourself, it's likewise significant not to be continually beating yourself up for not being at your actual weight as of now, in general, overheat because of stress, such self-recriminations will most likely cause you to feel even unhappier and significantly increasingly inclined to overeating—thus, the endless loop deteriorates.

So put forth an attempt to concentrate on those things you do like about yourself, and if you have days where you miss exercises or don't eat just as you'd like, be mindful so as not to blame yourself too brutally. Instead, recognize this is something that happens to everyone, and give a valiant effort to put it behind you and start anew merely. Recall that you don't need to eat or practice flawlessly to shed pounds—you need a moderate system that is sufficient.

If you can make these things part of your ordinary mindset, weight loss ought to be more straightforward. It tends to be somewhat testing, particularly in case you're accustomed to having a negative disposition towards yourself and your weight loss endeavors. One thing that can assist you with adopting a progressively empowered mindset all the more effective is to utilize a weight loss meditation recording. If you use a quality chronicle that incorporates brainwave entrainment innovation, you can increase more straightforward access to your subconscious mind and utilize necessary procedures, for example, affirmations and perception, to reconstruct it with new convictions that work for you as opposed to against you.

Such accounts contain dreary hints of specific frequencies, which make it simpler for your brain to enter a profoundly loose and centered state. In such express, the subconscious is increasingly open to the proposal, and any affirmation or perception work that you do will be progressively successful. That is an extraordinary method to assist with changing your mindset from the back to front, regardless of whether you're not knowledgeable about meditation or other mind control procedures. It's justified even despite the little exertion that it takes to do this since rolling out positive improvements throughout your life; for example, getting more fit is such a lot simpler when you have your mind on your side, battle your self-dangerous inclinations—because those desires aren't there anymore.

CHAPTER 13:

Script 4 – How Do I Love My Body If There Is No Reason?

These are all phrases that you should say to yourself as often as possible. As we read them, let them flow through your mind as if they are your own.

Write the words down to remember those further, put notes around your house with the affirmations written on them, or simply find other creative ways to incorporate these affirmations in your life. Let's start reading them now so that you can get these ideas in your head right away.

1. I have a happy and healthy attitude towards life.

2. I love my body; that is why I want the best for it.

3. I love myself; that is why I want to be healthy.

4. My health is my utmost priority.

5. My body is wonderful, and I love myself at the end of the day.

6. I can feel my body getting slimmer every day.

7. I can feel my appetite getting more manageable every day.

8. I believe in my capability to reach my goals of extreme weight loss.

9. Every day I weigh, the scales show significant weight loss.

10. Each day I successfully lose weight without fail.

11. My weight loss program is working like magic.

12. My body is responding immensely to my weight loss efforts.

13. I can feel my body fat melting away.

14. I have developed a high rate of metabolism that helps me reach my ideal weight.

15. I have complete focus on my weight loss journey.

16. Set a goal and achieve it.

17. Every day I wake up challenged and determined to reach my ideal weight goal.

18. Nobody can stop me from getting into the best shape of my life.

19. My determination to lose weight cannot be deterred.

20. My motivation to exercise is exceptional.

21. Every day I am motivated to follow a regular exercise regimen.

22. I am self-motivated and inspired to lose weight and follow a healthy lifestyle.

23. I already have a clear picture in my head of how sexy and beautiful/handsome I look when I finally reach my ideal weight.

24. Being healthy is not only a lifestyle for me but a principle that I am determined to keep.

25. I am choosing to be healthy and fit.

26. I choose to eat healthily and maintain an active lifestyle.

27. I choose to feel fit and sexy.

28. My mind is hard-wired to want only healthy food, and my body automatically feels that need for daily physical activity.

29. My mind only accepts positive thoughts and compliments about my body and resists any negativities that can divert me away from my weight loss goal.

30. I am surrounded by people who help and motivate me during my weight loss journey.

31. I feel grateful for my body and how effectively it responds to my weight loss efforts.

32. I am grateful for my strong will power and ability to manage my weight.

33. I am thankful for the people who are helping me reach my ultimate weight loss goals.

34. I divert myself from restaurants and establishments that can serve as a temptation to practice unhealthy eating habits.

35. I resist processed food, refined sugars, and salty snacks.

36. I have developed healthy eating habits.

37. I keep myself hydrated to aid in my weight loss.

38. I have established a regular exercise regimen that is very easy for me to follow.

39. I have embraced a life of clean and healthy living.

40. I have finally reached my ideal weight.

41. I am successful in my goal of extreme weight loss.

42. I invite all challenges that lead to a greater understanding of myself and my purpose.

43. My essence guides me daily toward better choices for my body.

44. I am blessed by the choices I make.

45. I am blessed by my ability to choose.

46. I have insights bestowed for my greater good.

47. I answer those insights with wisdom and enthusiasm.

48. I have used my intuition to develop sound confidence in my decisions.

49. I am what I have continuously thought and acted too.

50. I am the transformation the world needs right now.

51. I am the living embodiment of belief in action.

52. I use my body for exercise, my mind for belief, and my heart for forgiveness.

53. I have a choice to be who I want to be.

54. With that choice, I choose to let the flow of universal knowledge speak through me as a vessel of assertiveness.

55. I speak back to the universal flow with my actions.

56. I recognize those needs in all their usefulness, and I claim them for the roadmap to my self-appointed weight loss goals.

57. I am what I focus on.

58. I am the truth of my focus.

59. I love myself with a full heart.

60. I love my body with a full heart.

61. I love myself with a full mind.

62. I love exercising with a full spirit.

63. I am the love I need in my life.

64. I am healthy and my ideal weight.

65. I use my skills, knowledge, and resources to make the best food choices for my life.

66. I shine outward from within, and my body is an example of my inner beauty.

67. I welcome the challenge of exercise.

68. I welcome my sense of personal change.

69. I welcome my higher truth to speak through me.

70. I welcome my goals as benchmarks to help me achieve my ultimate level of happiness.

71. I boldly triumph over all obstacles.

72. I am thankful to receive these challenges to use my will to persevere.

73. I am appreciative of the challenges in my life for how they teach me to succeed.

74. I am successful because I have been tested and passed the tests with flying colors.

75. I am surrounded by teachers that offer me a chance to be my greatest self every day.

76. I am continuously thankful for my mentors, who show me how to overcome my doubts.

77. I am grateful for those who know my true worth and challenge me to see it in myself.

78. I move my body to eliminate stress.

79. I gravitate towards healthy decisions.

80. I rest my body after tireless effort.

81. I am the bravery I admire in others.

82. I move into that bravery with a warrior's spirit, ready for the challenges ahead.

83. That truth gives me the power to make wise choices.

84. I am the mountain.

85. I am the climber.

86. I put faith in my tools, for they assist me on my climb.

87. My motivation inspires my climb.

88. My tools assist me in my choice to persevere and succeed on my own.

89. I am the mountain I have conquered.

90. I am a warrior.

CHAPTER 14:

Preparing for Weight Loss

Weight loss affirmations are an extraordinary approach to move your excursion toward your weight loss. You can utilize these positive affirmations for getting more fit to help program your mind with positive propensities.

We all know that weight loss isn't almost that simple. We were utilizing these weight loss affirmations that can even assist the individuals who face obstinate inward obstruction when attempting to thin down.

Weight loss affirmations invite you. Here you will discover day by day affirmations for weight loss, which, whenever utilized regularly, will assist you with getting in shape.

Lasting weight loss or weight control requires an adjustment in the way of life. The affirmations given here will push you to change your way of life gradually.

Make astute and standard utilization of the positive affirmations for weight loss given underneath. As a rule, weight loss or weight control is an immediate capacity of our way of life.

The food we eat, the recurrence of eating, the method of consumption, the physical efforts that we experience, the rest we take, the psychological disposition that we keep up, all over an extensive period—in truth, over our total lifetime—decides our weight or potentially our weight issues. Utilize a reasonable weight-loss affirmation offered underneath to help with your concern.

Most diets work just as long as you work the diet! The other dieting stops, all the weight that has been lost gradually begins returning. This lone implies that except if you change your way of life, you will again have weight issues. Positive affirmations for weight loss will assist you in improving your way of life.

It has been discovered that our body keeps up the weight that our mind is OK with. If for reasons unknown, the brain thinks that it's vital. At that point, the body will begin collecting weight, and very before long will get itself overweight.

For instance, during youth, if you thought that it was useful to be "enormous bodied" for reasons of security, at that point, your subconscious mind will volunteer to make you huge and afterward to keep up your bigness. Weight picked up along these lines is hard to evacuate if the mind isn't managed first.

In such cases, no type of dieting will ever help. For substantial weight loss, it is essential to change our reasoning. You need to make your mind OK with the new weight you want. At times, heftiness is because of some glandular malfunction. In such cases, affirmations or diets may not work. You need to experience clinical treatment for the equivalent if you are overweight; at that point, counsel your doctor for any glandular issues before beginning a diet or affirmations.

Be cautious about the wording of the affirmation. Never state "I am not fat" because for this situation, you are concentrating on your concern, for example, being fat. Furthermore, whatever you center around, develops. Concentrate on the arrangement. So, the state should be, "I am thin" or "I am shedding pounds day by day and getting slimmer and slimmer."

Suppose you are a decided individual, at that point repeating the accompanying affirmations again and again, in any event, a hundred times day by day, ideally before a mirror, for a time of at any rate a half year. It will gradually assist you with taking a gander at and carrying on with an alternate life that is fitter than fatter. As usual, consolidate at least two of these free affirmations for weight loss, or even compose your sound weight loss affirmations, submitting a general direction to the accompanying.

Weight loss can appear to be difficult; utilizing weight loss affirmations to help you in the process can make it simpler. We should feel free to survey this large round to assist you with your weight loss venture.

1. Losing weight works out smoothly for me.

2. I am cheerfully accomplishing my weight loss objectives.

3. I am getting in shape each day.

4. I love to practice frequently.

5. I am eating nourishments that add to my well-being and prosperity.

6. I eat just when I am ravenous.

7. I now unmistakably observe myself at my optimal weight.

8. I love the flavor of healthy food.

9. I am pushing myself to work out; it causes me to feel great.

10. I am turning out to be fitter and more grounded regularly through exercise.

11. I am effectively reaching and keeping up my optimal weight

12. I love and care for my body.

13. I have the right to have a thin, sound, appealing body.

14. I am growing progressively good dieting propensities constantly.

15. I am getting slimmer consistently.

16. I look and feel incredible.

17. I take the necessary steps to be sound.

18. I am a joyfully re-imagined achievement.

19. I decide to work out.

20. I need to eat nourishments that cause me to look and to feel great.

21. I am answerable for my well-being.

22. I love my body.

23. I understand with creating my better body.

24. I am cheerfully practicing each morning when I wake up with the goal that I can arrive at the weight loss that I have been needing.

25. I am subscribing to my weight loss program by changing my eating propensities from unfortunate to sound.

26. I am content with each part I do in my extraordinary exertion to get in shape.

27. Every day, I am getting slimmer and more beneficial.

28. I am building up an appealing body.

29. I am building up a way of life of dynamic well-being.

30. I am creating a body that I like and appreciate.

Positive Affirmations for Losing Weight

1. My way of life eating changes is changing my body.

2. I feel incredible since I have lost more than 10 pounds in about a month and can hardly wait to meet my woman companion.

3. I have a level stomach.

4. I praise my power to settle on decisions around food.

5. I am cheerfully gauging 20 pounds less.

6. I am adoring strolling 3 to 4 times weekly and do conditioning practices, in any event, three times each week

7. Drinking eight bottles of water in a day.

8. I eat products of the soil everyday and taste, for the most part, chicken and fish.

9. I am learning and utilizing the psychological, emotional, and otherworldly abilities for progress. I will change it!

10. I will make new considerations about myself and my body.

11. I cherish and value my body.

12. It's energizing to find my one of a kind food and exercise framework for weight loss.

13. I am a weight loss example of overcoming adversity.

14. I am enchanted to be the perfect weight for me.

15. It's simple for me to follow a solid food plan.

16. I decide to grasp musings of trust in my capacity to roll out positive improvements throughout my life.

17. It feels great to move my body. Exercise is enjoyable!

18. I utilize deep breathing to assist me with unwinding and handle the pressure.

19. I am a delightful individual.

20. I have the right to be at my optimal weight.

21. I am an adorable individual. I merit love. It is ok for me to get more fit.

22. I am a solid nearness on the planet at my lower weight.

23. I discharge the need to reprimand my body.

24. I acknowledge and make the most of my sexuality. It's OK to feel arousing.

25. My digestion is impressive.

26. I keep up my body with ideal well-being.

27. I have faith in my capacity to adore myself for who I am.

28. I acknowledge my body shape and recognize the excellence it holds.

29. I am in charge of my future and the driver of my mind.

30. I let go of unhelpful examples of conduct around food.

31. I permit myself to settle on decisions and choices for my higher great.

32. I bring the characteristics of satisfaction, joy, and happiness into my life as I am currently.

33. I let go of any blame I hold around food decisions.

34. I acknowledge my body for the shape I have been honored with.

35. I let go of connections that are no longer for my higher great.

36. I have faith in myself and recognize my enormity.

37. I permit myself to feel great being me.

38. I acknowledge myself for who I am.

39. I bring the characteristics of adoration into my heart.

40. I have expectation and conviction about what's to come.

41. I am appreciative of the body I have and everything it accomplishes for me.

42. I weigh _____ pounds/kg.

43. Every day inside and out, I am moving toward my optimal weight.

44. I love being genuinely fit, and I lose enough weight with the goal that I am at my optimal weight.

45. My digestion rate is at its ideal, and it causes me to arrive at my optimal weight.

46. I love eating fresh food, and it causes me to arrive at my optimal weight.

47. I love practicing every day, and it causes me to arrive at my optimal weight.

48. I am a genuinely dynamic individual, and that encourages me to arrive at my optimal weight.

49. Every day inside and out, I am getting slimmer and fitter.

50. I appropriately bite all the food that I eat with the goal that it gets processed properly, and that encourages me to arrive at my optimal weight.

51. I inhale deeply without fail, so my digestion is at its ideal rate.

52. Every physical development that I make consumes the additional fat in my body and encourages me to keep up my optimal body weight.

53. I love myself unequivocally.

54. Life is lovely, and I appreciate life by remaining fit and keeping up my optimal weight.

CHAPTER 15:

Daily Mental Workout

This mental training allows you, every day, even for just a few minutes a day, to train your conscious and subconscious mind in the best way, and the best food intake condition.

In other words, with this mental training, you mentally project yourself in the best way of eating: slowly, taking small portions each time, chewing until each bite becomes liquid, remaining concentrated solely on the act of eating, and aware of the taste of food.

That is not a real self-hypnosis process, but a mental training performed in the self-hypnotic state, in which you will enter quickly. These allow you, with training, to reach the right state in a few seconds and to proceed with training even for a few minutes, several times a day.

What matters in this training, even more than in self-hypnotic sessions, is, in fact, repetition.

Repeat, repeat, repeat mental training. And then repeat it, repeat it, repeat it. And then repeat it, repeat it, repeat it until it becomes a habit and becomes an unconscious skill.

The secret is all here.

Use this hypnosis not as a step-by-step guided technique but as a basic recipe to be carried out independently: listen to it one or more times without training, then try to do it yourself, without listening to the audio, bring the skills acquired in any place and at any time, and activate training in any situation, whenever you want.

Sit comfortably.

Find a point of your choice in the room or place where you are to fix your gaze.

Fix that point without interruption.

You don't have to move your gaze even an inch. Just go back to fixing the chosen point immediately.

Look carefully at that point.

Continue to watch it carefully, without ever taking your eyes off it.

Feel how tiring it is for your eyes to keep them focused on that single point.

But keep doing it, without distracting yourself, even if your eyes get heavier.

The eyes can burn a little, blink slightly to let them rest, and just stare at that point.

The eyelids become heavier.

Keep looking at that point.

The eyelids become even heavier.

Keep looking at that point.

The eyes are tired, the eyelids drop.

Keep looking at that point.

The image of that point is blurred.

More and more.

The eyelids become even heavier.

More and more.

They are heavy as lead.

The eyes close with exhaustion.

Stay in this pleasant condition for a few seconds.

Then imagine that you are acting like eating.

Imagine eating when you are really hungry.

Imagine observing and smelling the dish with the meal.

Focus on perfumes.

Let yourself be filled with the scents of the food you are about to eat.

With cutlery, take a small portion of food and bring it to your mouth slowly.

Feel the taste of food.

Chew slowly.

Taste the food.

Continue to chew without haste without anxiety.

Continue to chew without feeling the need to swallow.

Continue to chew until the food in your mouth has become completely liquid.

Only then do you swallow.

Feel the food that gently descends into the body and brings health.

Feel the light digestion.

Between bites, always place the cutlery on the plate.

Keep repeating these actions for each bite and imagine eating until you feel full, put down the cutlery, move the plate away, and get up from the table.

Repeat these actions.

Repeat them, repeat them, repeat them.

That is what mental training consists of.

With training, your taste will become more and more sensitive, and you will always feel better the taste of each bite.

With training, you will learn to eat slower and eat less.

Mentally perform these actions without worrying about anything else: your subconscious will act to achieve it.

You can also use the technique to focus on specific aspects you want to improve and to strengthen self-hypnosis techniques. You can use mental training to continue to perceive the sense of satiety, or to refuse to eat compulsively, to eat calmly and serene, in full control and a state of well-being. And so on.

Use this mental training technique together with self-hypnosis techniques and as additional support for your real action on your food balance. And your real level of improvement will accelerate exponentially.

Important Tips for Performing Mental Training

The secret is to repeat, repeat, repeat by mentally performing the repetition to be already doing your best.

Don't worry if you don't seem to be able to imagine well or to visualize clearly: you don't have to worry. Repeat the sequences with confidence: your subconscious is perfectly processing your mental creation.

This mental repetition technique should be performed consistently every day. You can also perform it in cycles, giving yourself goals and periodically suspending it, and then resume it. Do it for a month, then pause, then resume for another month, and so on. Programming depends on you, but its secret, being progressive and parallel to your improvement, is continuous repetition—more continuity in the exercise, more continuity in success.

A final tip: try to perform mental training before your meals. Even if only for five minutes. In this way, you will undoubtedly remember the best actions throughout the meal to nourish yourself better, consciously, transforming each meal into a real exercise in health and well-being.

CHAPTER 16:

Weight Loss Affirmations

I n this chapter, we will learn about weight loss affirmations. They are a great way to stimulate your journey to weight loss. You can use these positive weight loss affirmations to program your mind with positive habits.

We all know that weight loss is not easy. The use of these weight loss affirmations can help people facing stubborn internal resistance when trying to lose weight.

These are the affirmations that you can suggest yourself while practicing self-hypnosis, cognitive-behavioral theory, or sleep learning system. In the first two methods, these affirmations can directly be suggested, and in the third method, you can record these and listen to them while sleeping.

You must be careful while choosing theses affirmations. You should select affirmations that you believe yourself and do not raise an objection when they are suggested to you. The failure happens because if you do not believe yourself, then it will not work for you. Moreover, it is suggested that you use a few affirmations that you think are effective for you. Do not try to suggest all at once. It may retard the effectiveness of the methods. There are also chances that the brain may become confused in case of any two opposite affirmations. So, better select your affirmations very carefully.

List of Affirmations for Excessive Weight Loss

1. Weight loss makes sense to me.

2. I want to reach the goal of weight loss.

3. I love to exercise regularly.

4. I eat foods that contribute to my health and well-being.

5. I only eat when I am hungry.

6. I can see myself clearly with my ideal weight.

7. I love the taste of healthy food.

8. I can control how much I want to eat.

9. I like training. I feel better.

10. Through exercise, I will be stronger and stronger every day.

11. I can reach the ideal weight and maintain it.

12. I love and care for my body.

13. I deserve a slim, healthy, and attractive body.

14. I always have a healthier eating habit.

15. I lose weight every day.

16. It looks good and feels good.

17. Whatever it takes, I need to be healthy.

18. I am happy to redefine success.

19. I decided to train.

20. I want to eat food that looks and feels good.

21. I am responsible for my health.

22. I love my body.

23. I put up with building a better body for myself.

24. When I wake up, I have a great time doing exercise every morning to achieve my desired weight loss.

25. I am working on a weight loss program by changing my diet from unhealthy to healthy.

26. I am happy with everything I do to lose weight.

27. I get thinner and healthier every day.

28. I am developing an attractive body.

29. I develop a lifestyle with life health.

30. I can create a body that I will like and enjoy.

These were general affirmations that you can use in a normal condition. You can move to more specific affirmations later when you feel that now it is time to modify my practice. Some of these affirmations that are given below will help you cope up with weight gain with a more specific approach.

1. Discovering my unique diet and exercise system for weight loss is exciting.

2. I accept and enjoy my sexuality. You can feel it sensually.

3. I am a beautiful person.

4. I am a weight loss success story.

5. I am happy to lose 20 pounds.

6. I am ready to develop new ideas about myself and my body.

7. I choose to trust the ability to make positive changes in my life.

8. I congratulate myself on choosing the right food.

9. I drink eight glasses of water daily.

10. I eat fruits and vegetables every day, mainly chicken and fish.

11. I enjoy walking 3-4 times a week and have at least three tonings exercised a week.

12. I free the need to criticize my body.

13. I have a strong weight in the world due to my low weight.

14. I learn and use mental, emotional, and spiritual skills for success. Ready to change!

15. I love and appreciate my body.

16. I will take care of my body in optimal health.

17. I'm happy that I have the ideal weight.

18. It feels good to move your body. The practice is fun!

19. It feels great to have lost more than 10 lbs in 4 weeks and can't wait to meet my girlfriend.

20. It's easy to follow a healthy diet plan.

21. My lifestyle changes my body.

22. My metabolism is excellent.

23. My stomach is flat.

24. Take a deep breath to relax and deal with stress.

25. My efforts are worth reaching the ideal weight.

You can make your affirmation to suit your routine and efforts. These affirmations in a normal routine or combined with methods that we discussed in this e-book can help reduce the weight quickly without affecting the emotional health.

CHAPTER 17:

Daily Affirmations

This segment will examine the importance of affirmations. An affirmation is something that you assert. It's a phrase stated factually, making sure that the information is understood. We frequently say affirmations to ourselves without thinking about it. You may consistently say to yourself, "I hate my activity." You may thoroughly consider it repeatedly, and before you know it, you're miserable and hating your activity because the thought affirmed that in your head daily. We have to flip affirmations around and use them to our advantage. Instead of consistently repeating negative things in your mind, aim to repeat positive phrases. We will talk about ways to remember affirmations for your daily lives. It takes minimal exertion to say these sentences, so actualize these strategies into your life ASAP.

The more you think these things, the more genuine they will feel, and the easier it will be to finish your weight loss goals. Saying these things will come naturally to you. We consider imagery a lot regarding our pattern of thought. If you're eager, you think, "I am starving," "I am wiped out," "I am not myself." These are dramatic statements, but they are topics that fly into our heads because that's how our brains are wired. We consistently connect thoughts to make sense of things. We also make absolute statements. You may fail once in a diet and think, "I can't do this." We create these assumptions because that's how our brains come up with an answer.

We must turn that intuition around and, instead, wire our brains to think entirely differently. To create your affirmations, speak in "I can," "I am," "I will," or "I have" statements. Use "I" in each affirmation you do, because this is all about increasing your positivity and creative reasoning, not for another person after you use the "I" phrases, next, move onto making a positive statement. Never depict what you lack, and attempt to avoid calling attention to your flaws, regardless of whether you are doing it decidedly. Speak in strong absolutes. The following four areas are examples of ones that you can use daily. Whichever area you battle with the most is the one you ought to incorporate the most affirmations from.

Motivational Affirmations

- I am a champ

- I am the most capable of completing the activity that I have to do

- I am not scared of failing

- Nothing that awaits me causes me to fear

- I have everything expected to take care of business

- I am more impressive than my greatest fear

- Each time I attempt I just get stronger

- I was made for something like this

- Giving up isn't in my nature

- My motivation is moving

- I have more motivation

- I am loaded up with motivation and the longing to continue onward

- The one in particular that is preventing me from the beginning is myself

- As soon as I start, I will already feel good

- I am ground-breaking

- I can complete whatever task

- I have done great previously so that I can improve going forward

- Finishing something always feels better than not doing it at all

- I am doing this because I can do it.

- I have no choices other than to start

- Getting started will be the greatest challenge

- There is nothing to fear other than not completing this task

- My knowledge is moving

- Making mistakes is natural, and I realize how to learn from them

- I take action when I realize I have to most

Weight Loss Affirmations

- My body is vigorous

- I love my body at any shape

- I feel the best when my body is healthy

- Taking care of my body feels better

- My body has gotten me through so much already

- My body is capable of anything

- I make healthy choices for my body

- I don't rebuff myself and just fill my mind with affection

- My mind feels clearer when I am concentrating on weight loss

- I do not care about the numbers; I care about how I feel

- All that matters is that I'm taking care of my body

- Losing some weight, regardless of how small, is better than losing none

- My life is better when I'm concentrating on my health and weight loss

- Losing weight will help me greatly in the long run

- I am taking care of myself now and later on

- Life is easier when I'm healthy

- I am getting the outcomes I've dreamt about

- Working hard to get thinner feels such better than fantasizing about it

- I love shedding pounds

- Every part of my body is healthy

- People appreciate how happy I am

- I love others more when I adore myself

- Being alive and healthy is something to be thankful for

- My body is marvelous

- I love the person I've become throughout my weight loss venture

Healthy Eating Affirmations

- Eating healthy feels better

- Eating healthy tastes great

- It is always better to fill me with something healthy

- The lousy nourishment I like isn't beneficial for me

- I allow myself to eat unhealthy once in a while, but realize that eating healthy takes priority

- Anything green hydrates me and keeps me full

- I am eating healthy for my entire body

- My heart feels full when I eat healthy foods

- Eating healthy reminds me I love myself

- Exercising is simple when I am eating healthy

- I am fortunate to have so much healthy food around

- I love trying various things with healthy food

- I am a superior cook when I make my healthy meals

- I always feel healthier whenever I eat healthily meals

- I don't realize all the advantages of eating healthy has on my body, until later on in the week

- My skin is shining because of the healthy foods I put in my body

- I don't have to eat unhealthy foods, because I realize that I feel good with healthy food in my body

- I don't have to fill my emotions with food

- Food makes me feel good, but healthy food encourages me to feel the best

- I need to eat to endure, so eating healthy is the way to satisfy this need, while also making me feel better

- I allow myself to enjoy now and again because I realize that garbage food can be useful for my mind sometimes

- I will always return to healthy food and make this my major core interest when cooking and preparing meals

- I am saving cash when I eat healthily

- I monitor my food when I eat unhealthily

- I drink water frequently

Self-Control Affirmations

- I am strong enough to realize how to say no

- I make sure that I say "yes" to doing the things that need to be completed

- I take care of my needs

- I strive to break terrible habits

- I am responsible for what I do

- Food doesn't have control over me

- Skipping my activities is just harming me in the long haul

- I am strong enough to know when I have to walk away from something

- I am sufficiently trained to begin

- I recognize what it takes to discover success

- I am in control of the things that come to me

- I am not afraid of a challenge

- I'm mentally ready to complete what I've started

- I am sufficiently strong enough to say no

- I am brave enough to begin all alone

- I buckle down because I merit the enormous payoff

- My self-control is motivating

- I am adept at completing things

- It feels so great to accomplish what I set out to do

- I am amazing

- I am strong-willed

- I am obstinate against myself

- I am my greatest inspiration

- I have been strong in the past and will continue to be into the future

- I am in control

CHAPTER 18:

Guided Meditation for Weight Loss

Meditation Exercise 1: Release of Bad Habits

Concentrate on your back now and notice how you feel in the bed or chair you are sitting in. Have a deep breath, and let your stress just go with the flow to leave your body. Now focus on your neck. Observe how your neck is joined to your shoulders. Lift your shoulders slowly. Breathe in slowly and release it. Feel how your shoulders loosen. Lift your shoulders again a little bit, then let them relax. Observe how your neck muscles are tensing and how much pressure it has. Breathe in and breathe out slowly. Release the pressure in your neck and notice how the stress is leaving your body. Repeat the whole exercise from the beginning. Observe your back. Notice all the stress and let it go with a deep breath. Focus on your shoulders and neck again. Lift your shoulders and hold it for some moments, then release your shoulders again and let all the stress go away. Sense how the stress is going away. Now, focus your attention on your back. Feel how comfortable it is. Focus on your whole body. While breathing in, let relaxation come, and while you are breathing out, let frustration leave your body. Notice how much you are relaxed.

Concentrate on your inner self. Breathe slowly in and release it. Calm your mind and observe your thoughts. Do not go with them because you aim to observe them and not to be involved. It's time for you to let go of that overweight self that you are not satisfied with. It is like your body is wearing a bigger, heavier top at this point in your life. Imagine stepping out of it and laying it on an imaginary chair facing you. Now tell yourself to let go of these old, established eating and behavioral patterns. Imagine that all your old, fixed patterns and all the obstacles that prevent you from achieving your desired weight are exiting your body, soul, and spirit with each breath. Know that your soul is perfect as it is, and all you want is for everything that pulls away to leave. With every breath, let your old beliefs go, as you are creating more and more space for something new. After spending a few minutes with this, imagine that every time you breathe in, you are inhaling prana, the life energy of the universe, shining in gold. In this life force, you will find everything you need and desire: a healthy, muscular body, a self that loves itself in all circumstances, a hand that puts enough nutritious food on the table, a strong voice to say no to sabotaging your diet, a head that can say no to those who are trying to distract you from your ideas and goals. With each breath, you absorb these positive images and emotions.

See in front of you exactly what your life would be like if you got everything you wanted. Release your old self and start becoming your new self. Feel the solid ground beneath you, open your eyes, and return to your normal state of consciousness.

Meditation Exercise 2: Forgiving Yourself

Sit comfortably. Do not cross your feet because this will lock you away from the desired experience. Hold your hands together to connect your logical brain hemisphere with your instinct. Relax your muscles, close your eyes.

Imagine a staircase in front of you! Descend it, counting down from ten to one.

You reached and found a door at the bottom of the stairs. Open the door. There is a meadow in front of us. Let us see if it has grass; if so, if it has flowers, what color, whether there is a bush or tree, and describe what you see in the distance.

Find the path covered with white stones and start walking on it.

Feel the power of the Earth flowing through your soles, the breeze stroking your skin, the warmth of the sun radiating toward you. Feel the harmony of the elements and your state of well-being.

From the left side, you hear the rattle of the stream. Walk down to the shore. This water of life comes from the throne of God. Take it with your palms and drink three sips and notice how it tastes. If you want, you can wash it. Keep walking. Feel the power of the Earth flowing through your soles, the breeze stroking your skin, the warmth of the sun radiating toward you. Feel the harmony of the elements and your state of well-being. In the distance, you see an ancient tree with many branches. That is the Tree of Life. Take a leaf from it, chew it, and note its taste and continue walking along the white gravel path. Feel the power of the Earth flowing through your soles, the breeze stroking your skin, the warmth of the sun radiating toward you. Feel the harmony of the elements and your state of well-being.

You have arrived at the Lake of Conscience, no one in this lake sinks. Rest on the water and think that all the emotions and thoughts you no longer need (anger, fear, horror, hopelessness, pain, sorrow, anxiety, annoyance, self-blame, superiority, self-pity, and guilt) pass through your skin. You purify them by the magical power of water. And you see that the water around you is full of gray and black globules that are slowly recovering the turquoise-green color of the water. You think once again of all the emotions and thoughts you no longer need, and they pass through your skin. You purify them by the magical power of water. You see that the water around you is full of gray and black globules that are slowly obscuring the turquoise-green color of the water. And once again, think of all the emotions and thoughts you no longer need as they pass through your skin, you purify them by the magical power of water. And you once again see that the water around you is full of gray and black globules that are slowly obscuring the turquoise-green color of the water.

You feel the power of the water, the power of the Earth, the breeze on your skin, the radiance of the sun warming you, the harmony of the elements, the feeling of well-being.

You ask your magical horse to come for you. You love your horse, you pamper it, and let it caress you too. You bounce on its back and head to God's Grad. In the air, you fly together, become one being. You have arrived. Ask your horse to wait.

You grow wings, and you fly toward the Trinity. You bow your head and apologize for all the sins you have committed against your body. You apologize for all the sins you have committed against your soul. You apologize for all the sins you committed against your spirit. You wait for the angels to give you the gifts that help you. If you cannot see yourself receive one, it means you do not need one yet. If you did, open it and look inside. Give thanks that you could be here. Get back on your horse and fly back to the meadow. Find the white gravel path and head back down to the door to your stairs. Look at the grass in the meadow. Notice if there are any flowers. If so, describe the colors, any bush or tree, and whatever you see in the distance. Feel the power of the Earth flowing through your soles, the breeze stroking your skin, the warmth of the sun radiating toward you. Feel the harmony of the elements and your state of well-being. You arrive at the door, open it, and head up the stairs. Count from one to ten. You are back, move your fingers slowly, open your eyes.

Meditation Exercise 3: Weight Loss

Sit comfortably. Relax your muscles, close your eyes, and breathe in and breathe out. Do not cross your feet because this will lock you away from the desired experience. Hold your hands together to connect your logical brain hemisphere with your instinct.

Concentrate on your back now and notice how you feel in the bed or chair you are sitting in. Take a deep breath and let your stress leave your body. Now focus on your neck. Observe how your neck is joined to your shoulders. Lift your shoulders slowly. Breathe in slowly and release it. Feel how your shoulders loosen. Lift your shoulders again a little bit, then let them relax. Observe how your neck muscles are tensing and how much pressure it has. Breathe in and breathe out slowly. Release the pressure in your neck and notice how the stress is leaving your body. Repeat the whole exercise from the beginning. Observe your back. Notice all the stress and let it go with a deep breath. Focus on your shoulders and neck again. Lift your shoulders and hold it for some moments, then release your shoulders again and let all the stress go away. Sense how the stress is going away. Now, place your attention on your back. Feel how comfortable it is. Focus on your whole body. While breathing in, let relaxation come in, and while you are breathing out, let frustration leave your body. Notice how much you are relaxed.

Concentrate on your inner self. Breathe slowly and release it. Calm down your mind. Observe your thoughts. Do not go with them because you aim to observe them and not to be involved. It is time to let go of your overweight self that you are not feeling good about. Imagine yourself as you are now. See yourself in every detail. Describe your hair, the color of your clothes, your eyes. See your face, your nose, your mouth. Set aside this image for a moment. Now imagine yourself as you would like to be in the future. See yourself in every detail. Describe your hair and the color of your clothes, eyes, face, nose, and your mouth and imagine that your new self-approaches your present self and pampers it. See that your new self hugs your present self. Feel the love that is spread in the air. Now see that your present self leaves the scene, and your new self takes its place. See and feel how happy and satisfied you are. You believe that you can become this beautiful new self. You breathe in this image and place it in your soul. This image will always be with you and flow through your whole body, and you want to be this new self. You can be this new self.

After spending a few minutes with this, imagine that every time you breathe in, you are inhaling prana, the life energy of the universe, shining in gold.

CHAPTER 19:

Using Affirmations for Weight Loss

An affirmation is just anything you state or think. We insist on what we expect in life all the time with our musings and convictions. The Universe, at that point, takes back to our encounters that coordinate the vibration of those considerations.

For instance, on the chance that you think discharging weight is troublesome and tiresome, it will be. If you trust it is trying now and again, however feasible, it will be. Your considerations about discharging weight make the nature of your excursion. They either assist you with succeeding or keep you down.

They are utilizing affirmations, just methods intentionally assuming responsibility for your musings. At the point when used with different methodologies, affirmations assist you with making a positive outlook for progress.

On the off chance that subliminal convictions are hindering your advancement, affirmations help kill them. Claims all by themselves, be that as it may, may not be sufficient to remove profoundly established or injury based convictions. These may best be settled through expert self-development work.

Saying positive affirmations doesn't mean you claim to feel energetic. The word positive likewise implies feeling certain and sure. At the point when you assert joyful musings, you reinforce your certainty to feel sure about accomplishing your weight reduction objectives. Notice what is avowed in these familiar ways of thinking about weight reduction:

"It's incomprehensible for me shed pounds."

"I've attempted previously, and nothing's made a difference. I don't perceive how this will be unique."

"It's difficult to get more fit when you're more established."

Do these words originate from somebody who will succeed or come up short? How about we turn these around:

"I can arrive at my weight reduction objectives."

"It doesn't make a difference what occurred previously; I will accomplish my objectives this time."

"Age has nothing to do with it. I can discharge this weight."

See the distinction? Here are some core values to utilize positive affirmations for discharging weight without hardly lifting a finger:

Discharge your connection to constraining convictions

You may hold convictions concerning why you figure you can't discharge weight. These convictions may originate from excruciating youth messages, for example, "You'll never add up to anything," or visually impaired concurrence with the cultural idea, for example, "Everybody knows it's hard to get in shape." Make space for positive affirmations to grab hold by opening your brain to supplant convictions that restrain you with elevating beliefs that help you. Utilize this fast check framework to decide whether a conviction aide or damages you:

"Does this conviction make dread or uncertainty?"

"Is this conviction despite my objectives?

If a conviction doesn't bolster you, change it.

Make affirmations that vibe regular to you

The intensity of affirmation increments when you put stock in them, and they are essential to you. Regardless of whether something doesn't yet feel valid, be that as it may, you can utilize affirmations to move toward whom you need to turn into delicately. For instance, on the chance that you state, "I discharge weight effectively," however where it counts you don't accept that, make an affirmation that feels genuine, for example, "I am available to discharge weight without any difficulty," or, "Although this feels troublesome on occasion, I am equipped for arriving at my objectives."

Use "I am" proclamations at whatever point conceivable

"I am" proclamations are especially incredible because whatever we connect to the words "I am," we become. There is a profound power within us, and it gives specific consideration to whatever follows our "I am" proclamations. So whether you state, "I am a disappointment" or "I am a triumph," you enact a strong force that delivers that outcome.

Use "I am" proclamations to mirror the characteristics you need, regardless of whether they don't yet appear valid. As you interface with the fantastic vitality inside you, in time, your "I am" proclamations will create the outcomes you want.

State affirmations in the current state

The Universe hears your musings and convictions truly and reacts in kind. Make affirmations that serve you right now and not in some future date. For instance, on the chance that you state, "I will get thinner," it keeps your advancement slowed down for some unsure future. However, if you state, "I am discharging weight," you confirm progress today.

Use affirmations when you feel loose and tranquil

Affirmations enter our inner mind all the more effectively when we're in a calm state. While it's essential to rehash claims for the day, make some calm time to extend their belongings.

A Daily Practice

Pick a few affirmations from the accompanying rundown. Change them to best suit you or make your own. Express your affirmations three to multiple times, or more, for the day.

You may think that it's supportive of keeping in touch with them on 3×5 cards to convey with you, add them to your PC foundation, or stay in touch with them on post-it notes put in apparent areas, for example, your washroom mirror or vehicle.

Make some calm time during the day where you can sit calmly, rehashing them.

State your affirmations with profound inclination, as though you, as of now, have the characteristics you're asserting.

Positive Affirmation Examples

Because of this definition, here are a few instances of positive affirmations:

- I have faith and belief in myself, and trust my shrewdness;

- I am an effective individual;

- I am sure and skilled at what I do.

Recorded underneath are progressively positive affirmation examples, concentrated on explicit territories.

9 Positive Affirmations for Women

Searching for certain plans to make your affirmations? Here are some pleasant examples:

- I decide to be upbeat;

- My life is occurring directly here, at this moment;

- I'm talented and encircled by astounding loved ones;

- I select to transcend negative emotions and jettison negative musings;

- I am versatile, hardy, and brave, and I can't be devastated;

- No one but me chooses how I feel;

- At the point when I have to rest, everything is as it ought to be, and I rest content;

- I am responsible for my contemplations, and I don't pass judgment on myself;

- I acknowledge and love myself, all together and totally.

9 Positive Affirmations for Men

Here are a few affirmations for men, including declarations of self-acknowledgment and positive self-perception. These affirmations depended on a more considerable rundown of 30 claims and were adjusted utilizing the intellectual, social treatment thought of "negative center convictions."

- I am answerable for taking care of me;

- By acting naturally, I carry bliss to others;

- My objectives and wants are as beneficial as everyone else's;

- Through mental fortitude and dangerous work, I can accomplish whatever I set my focus on;

- I'm fine with who I am, and I love who I am turning out to be;

- Through my commitments, I roll out positive improvements to the world;

- My body is astonishing only how it is, and I acknowledge myself along these lines;

- I pick just to encircle myself with steady and great individuals;

- At whatever point I tumble down, I get back up once more.

15 Positive Affirmations for Teens

Social weights and scholarly anxieties can negatively affect adolescents; however, they can pivot negative self-talk and accomplish something positive about what they think and feel. Here are a few affirmations that are appropriate for young people:

- I am a brisk, fit student;

- I have confidence in myself as an individual, and I put stock in all my abilities;

- I am one of a kind and delightful;

- Others regard me for following my convictions;

- On the off chance that a couple of individuals don't acknowledge me, I'm fine with that;

- I excuse others for now and then doing an inappropriate thing, and I pardon myself when I do likewise;

- I am benevolent and acceptable to the individual I find in the mirror;

- I have the right to consider myself to be stunning;

- Whatever troubles come to my direction, I can defeat them;

- I was brought into the world sound, and I develop more grounded each day;

- Today, I am going to confide in myself and my senses;

- I am adequate, and I am fine with only being me;

- I approach others with deference, and they treat me the equivalent;

- I decide to transcend the frightful things that may come to my direction;

- I am working each day on the best me that I can be.

11 Positive Affirmations for Kids

By figuring out how to rehearse positive affirmations at a young age, children can turn out to be substantially more arranged to utilize them when confronting troubles sometime down the road (Bloch, 2015). These are exceptionally straightforward affirmations because the more ignorant they are for little youngsters to recollect, the more probable kids will have the option to rehearse them without a grown-up's assistance.

- I am cherished;

- I am innovative;

- I am benevolent;

- I am fearless;

- I am a mindful individual;

- I will consistently give a valiant effort;

- I am interesting;

- At the point when I set out to accomplish something, I can do it;

- I'll generally help other people;

- I will adapt parts today since I am able;

- I am a significant and essential individual.

Ordinary Positive Affirmations for Students

Understudies may find that affirmations are useful for adapting to the pressure of scholarly life just as their extracurricular and public activities. Here are the examples from the full rundown that you or an understudy you know can use for inspiration or motivation.

- At the point when I get a terrible evaluation, I am persuaded to improve;

- I am resolved, and I focus on the stars;

- I set only requirements for my scholastic accomplishment. By investing energy and exertion, I can achieve what I set out to accomplish;

- I value my school, educators, and cohorts since they all assume a job in helping me develop as a superior individual;

- Indeed, even on days when I don't gain a lot of ground, I am continually learning. On different days, I get stunning ground toward my objectives.

6 Positive Affirmations to Help Relieve Anxiety

A great many people who have experienced nervousness will probably realize how significant it very well may be to cut off pessimistic idea designs before they start winding.

These affirmations can be utilized whenever, and even the individuals who don't commonly feel restless may discover them helpful during upsetting minutes.

During times of uneasiness or desperation, this rundown of positive affirmations can be utilized for consoling yourself. A couple of examples propelled by this asset include:

- I am freeing myself from dread, judgment, and uncertainty;

- I pick just to think great musings;

- My tension doesn't control my life. I do.

Some different affirmations identified with nonjudgment and care for nervousness can be found on this rundown. Here are some that draw motivation from the rundown:

- I inhale, I am gathered, and I am quiet;

- I am protected, and everything is acceptable in my reality;

- Inside me, I feel quiet, and no one can upset this tranquility.

CHAPTER 20:

Meditations for Positive Thinking and Self-Love

Often, we spend a lot of time worrying about loving other people. I want you to pause for a moment and ask yourself; do I love myself? Too often, we put ourselves behind everyone else, whether that be a child, a family member, or a significant other. I want you to realize that it's okay to put yourself first every once in a while. I want you to take a few moments right now to remind yourself how much you love you!

Having a positive mindset is one way to love yourself. While it may sound like a simple thing to do, it isn't always. When we have a positive mindset, this can help attract positive events into our life. It's much like the law of attraction like will always attract like. When you add positive thinking into your life, you will be able to attract positive things such as harmonious relationships and good fortune.

When you are ready, I would like to go through a few meditation scripts based around positive thinking and self-love. If you are having a rough day and are a bit down on yourself, I hope one of these scripts can help put a smile back on your face. Remember to live in the moment; you cannot be defined by your future or by your past. There is only now, and you have the power over how you feel about it.

Simple Smile Meditation Script

If you are having a rough day, you may have lost your smile. I want you to first begin by finding someplace that is comfortable for you. If needed, slip into some comfortable clothes or perhaps even wrap yourself up in your favorite comforter.

Once in place, I invite you to close your eyes gently and bring your attention to your breath. We will now go through a simple breathing exercise to help create a sense of serenity back to your mind and your body. Leave all of your issues at the door and focus only on your breath.

As you settle in, begin to breathe for four counts.

Inhale... four... three... two... one. Hold... four... three... two... one, and now exhale long and slow for eight counts... seven... six... five... four... three... two... one, wonderful.

Go ahead and repeat this process for a few more breaths. I want you to focus only on your breath and each number as it passes through your head.

Inhale... four... three... two... one. Hold... four... three... two... one, and now exhale long and slow for eight counts... seven... six... five... four... three... two... one, feel as your body is starting to let go of the tension, your mind becomes calm, your heartbeat becoming steady.

Inhale... four... three... two... one. Hold... four... three... two... one, and now exhale long and slow for eight counts... seven... six... five... four... three... two... one, great job.

When you are prepared to move on, go ahead, and bring attention to your face. Is there any tension that you can sense? Answer yourself kindly and allow for any judgments to pass without a second thought. Perhaps there is tension in your jaw, or your lips, or even behind your eyes. That is all perfectly normal, especially if you're not having the best of days.

While you become aware of these areas of tension, allow them to relax and soften. If you feel like it, allow your lips to form into a smile. As you do this, I want you to think of a family, friend, or a memory that you love dearly. Even if you have a hard day, there is always this person that can make you smile, even when you do not feel like it. I want you to take a few moments now to breathe and focus on this happy memory. Allow happiness to wash over you as you breathe.

As your smile becomes more natural, become mindful of how your heart is feeling when you are thinking of this memory. I want you to visualize what your heart is looking like right now, at this moment. Picture your heart pulsating and opening; it's beginning to spread love and positive energy all through your body. Take a few moments and focus on this love that is filling you up. When you are ready, I would like you to repeat it after me. We will be going over some positive affirmations that will hopefully place your smile back in place. Take another deep breath, and when you are ready, we can begin.

I can allow happiness to come to me.

(Pause)

I'm the only person in charge of my happiness.

(Pause)

I choose to smile, even in the hard times.

(Pause)

I'm happy and grateful for the life I lead.

(Pause)

When I choose to smile, others will smile with me.

(Pause)

I am truly happy and grateful.

(Pause)

If needed, you can repeat these phrases to yourself whenever you need them most. You truly are in charge of your happiness; no circumstance nor person can change that for you.

When you are ready, bring your awareness back to your breath. Notice now how much more relaxed your body feels and how a smile comes naturally back to your face. Gently bring your awareness to your space and gently give your body a little shake as you come back to the present moment. Allow your consciousness to awaken gently, smile, and you are ready to carry on with your day.

Guided Meditation for Self-Esteem Script

There are too many moments in our life when we are our own worst critics. If you are constantly bashing your body, putting yourself down, or feel you generally have low self-esteem, this script is going to be perfect for you! Through meditation, you can boost your confidence and your self-esteem. When you feel good about yourself, your body will be able to relax and just live life the way it's meant to be.

As always, I now invite you to relax. You will want to find your most comfortable position and allow all of the tension to begin melting away from your limbs. As you find your breath, I want to paint a picture for you. Simply do nothing right now but allow for your breath to become natural.

As you breathe, I want you to picture a staircase in your mind. Right now, you are standing at the top of these stairs. As you look down at the bottom, there is a pool of relaxation and peace. When you are looking down, I invite you to take a mental note of how you are feeling right now.

Take a deep breath and picture yourself taking a soft step down. With this step, you are already closer to the relaxation pool you want to be floating in. Each step you take down, feel how much more relaxed your body is becoming. Your arms are relaxing; your legs are relaxing; your jaw is becoming loose as you step closer and closer to the bottom of the stairs.

One step at a time, you are making your way down the stairs. Your arms are feeling heavier, your legs are heavier, the relaxation is pulling you down gently, and it feels comfortable. You are safe at this moment, and slipping into the pool of relaxation will be such a relief. Allow for gravity to pull you down gently.

Feel now as your back and your neck are both relaxing, too. Your shoulders being pulled away from being shrugged up into your shoulders, your eyes becoming heavy with relaxation, and every part of your body is becoming calm and relaxed. Go ahead and allow for your mind to drift away from you. Everything is feeling wonderful as you approach the bottom of the stairs.

Now, you are taking the final steps to the bottom of the stairs. Go ahead and admire the pool of relaxation as you gently step in. Allow for your mind to drift as you settle into the calmness of the pool and rest your eyes. Your whole body is loose and relaxed; you haven't a care in the world.

I would like you to allow your mind to drift now. As it does, I would like to go over some positive affirmations for your self-esteem. You can listen to them and repeat them if you would like to. While some may apply to you, others may not. Listen to your mind and your heart as we go over the affirmations. Once we are done, you can allow your mind to continue drifting. Simply breathe, relax, and we can begin.

You are capable of doing so many amazing things with your life.

You are a loving person, and you deserve to be happy.

You are strong, but you do not need to be strong all of the time.

You are worth it.

You have the power to control your emotions.

It's okay to accept yourself.

You need to be kind to yourself.

You are perfect the way you are at this moment.

It's okay to be happy.

It's okay to be proud of yourself.

Now, repeat after me.

I'm capable of doing so many amazing things with my life.

I'm a loving person, and I deserve to be happy.

I'm strong, but I do not need to be strong all of the time.

I'm worth it.

I have the power to control my emotions.

It's okay to accept myself.

I need to be kind to myself.

I'm perfect the way I am at this moment.

It's okay to be happy.

It's okay to be proud of myself.

Allow for your mind to drift and repeat these affirmations as needed. You can repeat them until you believe them. These are all true for you, and you deserve to build your sense of self-assurance and confidence. You will always have yourself. It's up to you to become your biggest cheerleader!

You can, and you will make positive changes in your life. When you increase your self-esteem and gain a positive mindset, you will begin to attract positive events and positive people into your life.

Now, I want you to bring awareness back to your mind. Feel now how much happier and relaxed you feel. Notice how calm you are and take a moment to enjoy this new sensation. Any time you are feeling down on yourself, I want you to repeat these affirmations to yourself. You deserve to feel good. Be in charge of your happiness.

When you are ready to return to your day, take a few more deep breaths. Gently bring your awareness back to your space and return to your day with positivity and gratitude.

Positive Body Image Script

Let's face it; there is always something that we don't approve of on our bodies. I'm here to tell you that you need to stop being so hard on yourself! Everyone else out there is judging you, stop being mean to yourself. You have a heart in your chest, you have lungs that keep you breathing, and you have a body that allows you to get through life. It's time to appreciate everything that you have instead of fretting over the things you don't.

The body cannot function properly without enough sleep. It will affect other organ systems in your body. Stress and sleeplessness may lead to a more severe problem, and other mental health issues may occur. The solution to this problem may be deep sleep hypnosis.

CHAPTER 21:

Meditation for a Mindfulness Diet

Visualization, suggestion combined with meditation, is an easy way to make positive and powerful personal changes. If you combine meditation with positive affirmation, you will begin to change the way you feel, think, and act. This relaxation exercise will help you change and improve the way you feel. However, time is taken to see the effects that differ from person to person. Let's begin.

Sit or lie down comfortably.

Stretch your back, and then put your shoulders backward to open the rib cage.

Feel your shoulder muscles relax.

Close your eyes.

Relax your body and empty your mind.

Take ten slow but deep breaths.

Concentrate on the breath.

Feel it getting slower and deeper.

Feel relaxed as every tension goes away.

Relax your neck and shoulders again.

(Pause a minute for reflection)

Imagine being happy, being successful, winning, being loved, laughing, feeling good.

Relax your forehead, mouth, and eyes.

Let a soft smile appear on your face as you feel a calm enter your mind.

(Pause a minute for reflection)

(Meditation closing)

Then say the following words:

I'm a good person.

I do what is right.

I have integrity.

Whatever life presents is a useful experience that will only make me wiser, stronger, and more tolerant.

I eat and drink good things.

I am what I eat and drink.

I focus on the joy in my life.

I am what I see, touch, and hear positive things.

I am compassionate, loving, and caring.

I am strong enough to understand that the behavior of others is about them, not me.

I help others when I can.

I exercise because I enjoy it.

I smile and laugh because I am happy.

I help other people. After all, they are all good people, like me.

I'm what I say I am.

I am.

Meditative affirmations are a centuries-old way of gaining control over our feelings and behaviors.

Meditation for Positive Thinking

This hypnotherapy experience will allow you to fall asleep easily. At the same time, your calm and relaxed mind can enjoy listening along to a series of beneficial suggestions, all of which are in the form of positive affirmations to enhance your health, wealth, and happiness.

You will find that there is nothing overly complicated in this session. Allow yourself to drift into hypnosis and then away into your dreams.

During this relaxing time ahead, your conscious mind will inevitably wander, but your subconscious mind will continue to listen to my voice.

As you settle in and lay your head on the pillow, you can be reassured that all of these suggestions will speak powerfully to your subconscious mind. It makes no difference whether you remember or forget the pleasant suggestions in this session. You can trust in my voice to permeate your subconscious being while you fall into the deep state of hypnosis.

As you are preparing to relax, take a moment to reassure yourself that all hypnosis is self-hypnosis, which means that you remain in control throughout the entirety of this session. If something from the outside world requires your presence at any time, you can simply open your eyes, and the hypnosis will be over.

But for now, you can continue to relax and allow the noise and distractions of the outside world to continue to fade away gently into the night.

Because this time is the perfect time to let go and let it all drift away

That is the perfect time to relax

If they aren't already, close your eyes lightly.

Throughout this time, there is no need to do anything. There is no need to worry about things that happened today or things that might happen tomorrow. Right now, all you need to do is to be here, in your body, on your bed, letting your mind do what it needs to do to relax for a good night's sleep.

Thank you for taking this time for self-care. You deserve a night of restful sleep and to wake up feeling refreshed and ready for the day. That is one thing that you can do that is just for yourself. No guilt, no worries.

Know that whatever worries you and stops you from sleeping won't be fixed by keeping you awake.

Know that no matter how you slept last night or the night before, you can sleep well tonight. That is the only night that matters.

Just let yourself go.

Lie still as you allow the stress to fade away.

(Pause a minute for reflection)

Each time you find your mind drifting, notice where it's gone and gently tell yourself to come back to being right here, right now. There is no need to judge what your mind is thinking about or that you have become distracted. That is what our brains are designed to do.

Now, take a deep breath.

And exhale.

Take a deep breath.

And exhale.

Take a deep breath and feel the air as it flows through your nostrils, down into your lungs, and fully into your abdomen. Breathe in as deeply as you can.

(Pause a minute for reflection)

As your body relaxes, it may begin to feel heavy. Feel how it rests on the bed. You are supported in this meditation by the things around you. They hold you and allow your mind to do the work needed to unclutter your mind.

Like your breath, your body may hold areas of tension that distract you. When you notice tension, try to relax those muscles. You may find that a small stretch and release of the muscles help reduce the tension. That doesn't have to be a big movement. Just enough to allow your muscles to fall back down into a restful state.

That is something that resets the muscle memory into one of relaxation rather than tension.

Now, take a deep breath.

And exhale.

Deep breath.

And exhale.

(Pause a minute for reflection)

Now, I will count down from 10 to 1.

With each passing number, you will feel yourself falling deeper and deeper into a peaceful state of relaxation.

With each passing number, you will feel your body grow increasingly heavier. Allow this feeling to wash over you, and allow the tension from your muscles to fade away. Allow yourself to relax.

10.

9.

8.

7.

6.

5.

4.

3.

2.

1.

I am learning to relax to the deepest I can go.

I am learning to relax to the deepest I can go.

With each breath, I fall deeper into a state of relaxation.

With each breath, I fall deeper into a state of relaxation.

I slowly release all control.

I slowly release all control.

(Pause a minute for reflection)

(Meditation closing)

I am the architect of my life.

I am unique.

I am happy.

I am successful.

I am positive.

I am special.

I am in full control, relaxed, and comfortable.

I am now in the perfect place, and this is the perfect time to rest and sleep.

I welcome dreams of positivity and abundance.

I welcome relaxation with a heart full of gratitude.

With each breath, I dive deeper into a state of relaxation.

With each breath, I dive deeper into a state of relaxation.

Positive energy comes to me easily and effortlessly.

Positive energy comes to me easily and effortlessly.

The more I let go, the deeper I relax.

The more I let go, the deeper I relax.

Meditation to Cope during Difficult Times

Sit comfortably with your legs crossed and your arms placed on your thigh's palms facing up.

(5 seconds)

Take three deep breaths and exhale completely with each breath.

(30 seconds)

Keeping your breathing deep will allow your body to become relaxed.

(60 seconds)

Now, bring your attention to the challenges you are facing. Without thinking too much about them, just identify them one by one.

(20 seconds)

How are you feeling? Are you mad, sad, stressed, in pain, or sorrowful? Identify the emotions that stand out for you at this moment.

(10 seconds)

Realize that these emotions are a manifestation of the chemical process taking place in your body. Therefore, notice them without judgment or getting involved in them.

(15 seconds)

Do not try to push them away either. Instead, become a curious observer. Notice how intense they are. Are they manifesting on a specific part of the body? For instance, can you feel heaviness at your solar plexus, or do your shoulders feel tight? Is your heart feeling a bit faster? Have you lost your smile and your jaw is tightly clenched and lips tightly closed? Become aware of the parts of the body that these emotions are manifesting.

(30 seconds)

Whatever feelings you are experiencing, you do not need to be ashamed of them just because you perceive them as negative feelings. Be open to them. See them as a way of your body responding to various circumstances and happenings. It is all right, you are human, and you are allowed to feel how you are feeling at this moment.

(60 seconds)

Now, begin to deepen your breaths.

(20 seconds)

Take notice of your hands and tighten them into fists.

(5 seconds)

Make the fists tighter and notice tension build up in your hands.

(5 seconds)

Release the tight grip on your fists and allow your entire hand to become limp.

(5 seconds)

Become aware of your shoulders.

(5 seconds)

Think of how they would feel if they were relaxed. Now, tighten the muscles around the shoulders and then relax them.

(20 seconds)

Take your attention to your face.

(5 seconds)

Narrow your focus to your jaw. Tense your entire jaw. Now allow the jaw to relax and notice as the tension melts away.

(5 seconds)

Now scan your whole body and search for hidden stress in the muscles. Relax every area that you can sense tension.

(120 seconds)

Scan one more time to see if there is any part of the body that is still tensed even if just a little bit. Tighten the body part and allow it to relax.

(60 seconds)

Now scan the whole body from your head to your toes. Take a deep breath in and tightly squeeze all the parts of your body. Hold your breath in and continue to squeeze your muscles some more. Begin to exhale as you relax the entire body.

You are no longer hiding these emotions.

You have taken a step to allow yourself to feel them, but not giving them control over your life.

Remember that allowing yourself to acknowledge these negative feelings is an act of courage.

(10 seconds)

Once again, begin to take deep breaths.

(20 seconds)

With the expansion of every inhale, allow your body to create room in your heart for positive emotions. With the contraction of every exhale, become aware of your ability to cope with difficult times and emotions.

(5 seconds)

Keep breathing in and out as you allow your body to create more space for grace, strength, and courage.

(60 seconds)

Now, allow your breathing to adapt to its normal rhythm and just observe it.

(60 seconds)

Think of a time when you were delighted and at peace. When was it? How was life then? How did you feel? Remember that moment in detail.

(20 seconds)

Allow yourself to relive that moment, and for the emotions, you felt then to fill your body and mind.

(20 seconds)

CHAPTER 22:

Return to Happiness by Loving Your Body and Healing Your Soul

Glad individuals acknowledge and love themselves regardless of what their body resembles, regardless of how they feel. An ideal body isn't preferred or all the more empowering over a body not considered immaculate by the "powers that be." Your magnificence originates from inside.

Consider somebody you know (or knew) who isn't generally all that appealing; however, who appears to adore herself so much that she feels delightful and acts as needs to be. Individuals like that tend to be well known. Curiously, their excellence sparkles so splendidly that they seem, by all accounts, to be alluring to others.

What is your opinion about your body shape? What about your body condition? How is your well-being? Is it true that you are happy with your physical and emotional well-being?

Imagine a scenario in which your body doesn't fit the portrayal of lovely, as indicated by the media. Does that cause you to feel not exactly second rate or ugly? Who sets the incredible gauges for the media?

Individuals in the media don't typically seem as though they seem to look in front of an audience or magazines and films. That is the reason the calling of make-up specialists exists. In my mind, what they do is makeup how this individual will appear to the crowd and fans. When photograph distributing is included, nobody is viewed as they look. All photographs get finished up.

To whose norms do you hold yourself? Consider the possibility that something about you changes. At the point when you discover and characterize your excellence inside, then nothing in your outside world changes how you feel about being you—nothing.

At the point when you love yourself, truly and genuinely love yourself, regardless of how old you develop to be, your sentiments about you won't change. The fascinating piece about adoring yourself is living in a condition of satisfaction. Hardly any individuals get the chance to abide there—the individuals who do remain youthful until the end of time.

Coincidentally, would you like to get familiar with how you can live in bliss now?

Figuring Out How to Love Your Body

Ordinarily, we are assaulted with pictures of models with impeccable bodies. That can be terrible for our self-regard. How might we figure out how to cherish our bodies when we are continually being contrasted with these incredible immaculate bodies? All things considered, or starters, don't stress over what individuals think a solid body is directly for you.

To begin with, you should work out. Research has demonstrated that practicing routinely will help your self-regard. Isn't it so extraordinary? You won't just have a more advantageous trimmer body, yet you will likewise feel incredible about yourself. So, get out and exercise and consume those calories. You don't have to go to the exercise center; you can do it at home, busy working, or outside.

As referenced before, we are encircled by these pictures of models with alleged impeccable bodies. There is nothing of the sort! We, as a whole, ought to have a body that we're agreeable in. Acknowledge your body shape and spotlight on how you can get more advantageous, and that is simply the ideal approach to figure out how to cherish yourself.

The choice is in your grasp. Pardon me for saying this. You can say that you're content with being fat and can acknowledge yourself as a husky individual. However, can you truly? Genuinely? Would you truly like to be unfit, unfortunate, and drowsy constantly? So, take a gander at the advantages and disadvantages, and you'll see that getting fit and sound is consistently the better choice. Once more, and I feel compelled to pressure this as much as possible, be consistent with yourself. You shouldn't resemble the supermodels to be exceptional. You are an interesting individual with great qualities. So, center around that, and you will before long observe that the more benefits you have, the more joyful you will be. When you figure out how to adore your body, you will see that you are more joyful with yourself, and you presently carry on with your existence with an increasingly uplifting disposition. Figure out how to acknowledge your body type, get ordinary exercise, and eat a sound diet, and you will see an extraordinary improvement satisfaction.

Five Ways to Love Your Body and Get Fit as a Fiddle

The strain to get fit and sound is in high rigging. Individuals are anxious to locate the ideal approaches to put themselves on the road to success to well-being and bliss. One misstep that numerous individuals are making anyway is ignoring their body's fundamental needs as they proceed with their journey for that ideal physical make-up. You need to address your physical, emotional, and profound necessities during your excursion to better wellness and the reason you need to figure out how to cherish your body and praise the experience of being **you!**

Adoring your body implies that you can grasp the magnificence existing apart from everything else and acknowledge who and where at present. At the point when you can do this, it will empower you to discover fulfillment and joy at each phase of your workout schedule.

Here are five different ways to adore your body now and begin headed straight toward better well-being:

Lower the Boom on Stress

Stress is probably the greatest foe of your mind and body. Regardless of how seriously you are working out, if you are keeping up elevated levels of pressure, your activity and wellness routine will be disrupted. Lessening pressure is a key component that will show your body you truly care.

Yoga and meditation are two strategies that numerous individuals have discovered successful in countering pressure. It may not have a difference as regards what you pick as a way to dispose of the stressors throughout your life as long as it is an action that makes you glad and truly facilitates the distressing requests on your mind and body.

Better Nutrition

You have heard these multiple occasions previously, however, even though everything bears repeating. Your food decisions have a ton to do with how your body looks, feels, and reacts to insightful choices about the nourishments that you will eat. Fuel your body with the freshest veggies and organic products.

Hurl out those over handled low-quality nourishments and arranged meal bundles, find the delight of good dieting, and show your body that you truly care.

Work Out with Weights

Exercise is terrifically significant with regards to cherishing your body. The total workout program ought to include oxygen-consuming and anaerobic exercises. You should likewise join weights into your ordinary exercise schedule. Not exclusively will working out with weights consume fat and assist you with getting more grounded; it assembles bone quality, which is an extraordinary reward for your body.

Set Aside Effort for You

Somewhat self-spoiling is a need, not an extravagance. At any rate, once per week, you have to put aside an hour or two just to entertain yourself. An invigorating back rub with hot stones is an ideal method to loosen up. Those tight muscles and hurting joints will be restored, and you will find that you unexpectedly have a "renewed purpose for carrying on with life." A loosening up spa day at a neighborhood salon is, in every case, great, yet you can simply absorb a tub of warm water at your home. Set the state of mind with candles, blossoms, and fragrant oils, and you will rapidly observe the constructive outcome this loosening up time has on your mind and body.

Accept Circumstances for What They Are

Maybe the ideal way you can show your body the amount you love is by turning out to be sensitive to the signs that it gives. You have to tune in to these signs when you are starting any exercise or exercise schedule. Try not to request beyond what your body can give. Find a steady speed as you manufacture your quality and endurance. Try not to contrast yourself as well as other people because your body is novel. Recollect that getting fit as a fiddle is a long-distance race work in progress, and it's anything but a 24-hour run. Take things at a sensible pace and permit yourself to accept the way things are. You will arrive at the end goal in top structure if you work with your body rather than against it, and isn't this a genuine demonstration of affection?

For what reason do you love your body? Do you love your body since, as Beth expressed above, it houses your radiant soul? Do you love your body since it empowers you to encounter the wealth of existence with the entirety of your faculties? Do you love your body since it permits you to make things, embrace others, and appreciate the joy of development? We need to begin the discussion about cherishing your body with the why not the if—to get you to move your speculation toward that path right away. Individuals, ladies specifically, maybe you, the peruse—have spent fearfully numerous valuable snapshots of life condemning and attempting to change your body instead of genuinely adoring and tolerating the endowment of your body!

The test that most ladies face around adoring their bodies is the social molding around the perfect body for ladies. There was a famous advertisement for "The Body Shop," the skin and hair care items organization, which expressed, "There are 3 billion ladies who don't seem as though supermodels and just eight who do." This promotion featured that what is advanced as the perfect, typical body for ladies is the ordinary body for just an extremely little level of ladies. However, this picture is constantly depicted in publicizing, on magazine covers and, in the entertainers, we find in films and on TV.

It is a twisting of reality that winds up creating a circumstance where ladies feel lacking and that there is some kind of problem with their body for not resembling this. It makes ladies judge and attempt to change their bodies by dieting, plastic surgery, and numerous different methods of attempting to get their bodies to resemble the perfect. This social molding is frightful and harms ladies and young ladies. It is poisonous because rather celebrating and adoring their special shape, and they are making a decision about it against the advanced perfect. As per the Social Issues Research Center, "Over 80% of fourth-graders have been on a prevailing fashion diet." It is miserable to see the weight that little youngsters feel to begin to form their bodies into the perfect, as opposed to utilizing this vitality to learn, investigate and simply be cheerful and content acting naturally.

CHAPTER 23:

Self-Image – Weight Loss

By self-esteem, we talk of body image in particular. When people have a bad picture of themselves, it feeds back into the emotional part. The bad the body image of someone, the less likely they are to adopt a healthy lifestyle. Why? Why? There are a few explanations for this. One is embedded in the feeling: "Why bother? My body is ugly, it's awful, it's still my enemy, why should I bother trying to take care of it?"

And then in this kind of thinking, there is ignorance:

"Oh, even I don't know what is happening. I'm so scared of my body, I don't like how it looks, and I don't know, so right now I will go for good and not just good, but in half an hour."

Most positive emotions add up to a very unhealthy lifestyle right now. When someone's view of the body is out of control and seeks to dissociate them from their bodies, the food aspect is less important. Interestingly, they're not hunting for healthier products, so it just doesn't matter. It's a shame they're struggling to feel better right now.

Let's now look at someone who has a healthy body and a healthy self-image, spiritual or not.

When they are spiritual, a very simple reframe can be used along the lines:

- "You gave this body some stronger or more strength from above. It's your ride. You may want to know how to care for it."

One sort of reframing is the whole concept that your body is your temple. The notion that the body is the main interface with the world can also act as a legitimate reframe for people who have not been similarly inclined. It's like a connection to the internet. Similar to high-speed broadband, if you have a sluggish dial-up modem, it is easy to say the difference. The same is true for the life experience of your subject.

The more you are in touch with your food and physical needs, the more your brain and mind function, and the greater your life experience. You do not have to deal with it. In other words, don't repair it if it's not broken.

One way of finding out whether there is the problem is to ask a set of near-magical questions:

- What do you feel when you look into the mirror?

- Have you ever seen yourself in the mirror of the shower in the nude? Why do you see what you're seeing?

- What do you see at the moment? Describe yourself.

These questions are almost magical because they evoke an answer. Listen in their descriptions to words and especially adjectives. They are likely to have an issue with their self-image if they use derogatory words such as "horrible, gross, bad, unsafe, nasty." You probably have a good self-image if you use overall compassionate words.

You must always pay attention to your emotional tone and features. The vocabulary may be inherently sympathetic, but if the emotional tone is repulsive, for instance, then a secret decision is probably made. You may be socially friendly by saying what you think you want to hear; however, your feelings will betray you.

How to Help People Improve Their Self-Image

There are two main self-image components. The first is sympathy for oneself, and the second is the prejudice of affirmation. Let's deal with these individuals.

Self-compassion is about being good to you. Knowing you're good enough, you're all right. Self-compassion starts where you are from. And if you make poor decisions, you don't want to punish yourself. When you do, cognitive dissonance is formed. Those times you're not going to want to think about because they feel bad. It means you're not going to benefit from them, and the chances are high to repeat them. If it gets very bad, you will manifest a part of yourself that binge eats to punish you.

The bad behavior comes out, and you don't control it. That is more like having an alter ego that eats the binge. That is avoided by self-compassion. It helps it to go. You know you made a bad choice of food and binged, but it's all right. Forgive yourself. You're going to do great tomorrow. And that's the next day.

Feeling caring for yourself doesn't mean you let go. That just means you can make mistakes from time to time. The opposite side is a validation distortion. Whenever you feel bad about your body, you can believe that it is worse than it is. A behavior is: what is the point? You let yourself go, and you become that very thing.

You can hear them say, for example, "Look, I eat well. I am still obese. I'm still overweight. I'm still unattractive."

You want to prove yourself correctly. That is the prejudice of belief and one of the psychological effects most difficult to resolve.

Naturally, methods like the classical double-blind language and another mind-altering language can be used.

When a person has an awful self-image, you might ask them:

- "Which body part do you want? Pick just the part of your body that you like even a little."

- "What part of your body would you say is maybe the nicest?"

- "How much do people compliment you; on what part(s) of your body?"

What are they going to say? Who knows? Yet something they're going to have to claim. You will pick one part of your body. You'll assign them a mission then. Suppose your favorite physical feature is your smile. Tell them to note their smile in the following week and then tell you how much they smile.

What you do is continue to use a confirmatory bias to guide you towards the quantities of stuff you like about your body.

It is the old classic Ericksonian double-blind: which one of your hands now feels lighter?

Which one of your hands now feels most unusual?

The fact that they respond means that they are looking for some kind of information. You search for proof.

You may even ask them to remember which part of their body shocked them, so they like it more than they know.

It is the language of mind-bending at work. You're going to get curious about your body in a way that your connection to your body image searches for things that work.

Let's assume, for starters, that they're overweight. You have other medical conditions as it affects your breathing, your pulse, and your cholesterol levels. No, they haven't got diabetes. It is really important for the reframe below.

You tell me that you are putting all this thing in your body and that, as a result, your body has reached that condition, but you have no diabetes. What did your body manage on earth to keep diabetes away while most people have it? That is a good job. How is your body doing such a good job on earth? It is the secret to self-image to find what they do correctly.

If they're still alive, something's right. If they didn't do anything wrong, then they would have another question. They will be dead, and for that, there's no cure. When you have learned to despise your body early in life, you might continue to relapse and repress.

You may have to make a series of regressions to retrain them to learn how they respond to their bodies. When you like the sound of your voice, you have to know that your body produces the sound.

You can, therefore, thank them. You may revive your singing and your speech and wonder how your body creates it. And what a wonder your body is. That is a powerful Ericksonian trick that tells them that their bodies are unique. It's an amazing creature. When someone starts appreciating his body as an amazing tool, they'd like to take better care of it—a guy who loves his car.

They keep it tidy, tidy, and suspicious, particularly with food or drink, when someone comes too close to it. You appreciate that. And what if everyone decided to care about their body in the same way?

People who love their car do not put in cheap fuel or gasoline. It's their kid. I love it. We love it. And they carefully surround it with the finest materials to hold it in top condition. If someone were to relate to their body with the same sensation of wonder as a car enthusiast, they would like to take extra care of it.

It is the core of the process' self-image, to make them enjoy their bodies again, to see the magic of it.

You can do this with basic facts about your body, which contribute to a confirmatory distortion.

You teach a mentality that eventually leads them to believe their body is a wonderful thing worth taking care of.

CHAPTER 24:

The New Behavior Generator

Have you ever start doing something that would be valuable or resourceful to you? Is it changing your eating patterns? Is it doing your yard work?

I am notorious for having the second-worst yard on my block. I never want to be the worst yard in the neighborhood; I have just never been a big fan of doing yard work before. I have no problem being the second-worst yard in the neighborhood: I don't get all the negative attention, and I don't have to expend energy to make my yard look nice.

Last year I bought a new house. When I bought the new house, I decided that I was going to, after 50 some years, finally break the mold of having the second-worst yard in the neighborhood and take care of my yard. I bought a hedge trimmer. I bought a weed eater. I bought some buckets to pick up debris. I bought a blower. I bought a big broom. I bought all the accouterments that I would need to be able to take care of my yard and perhaps be able to bump myself up to the owner of the best yard in the neighborhood.

Even though that was my intention when I moved in, I noticed after a few months of living there that I had, once again, returned to my old title of the owner of the second-worst yard in the neighborhood.

So, what I did was the self-hypnosis technique called a New Behavior Generator. It is amazing! Whatever new behavior you would like to generate, you can use this strategy to do so. It will program you to not only act on the behavior but to make it a habit. Park with the kids and our golden doodle, I pulled into my driveway, and I looked at my yard.

I was proud of my yard, realizing that my yard was way better than most of my neighbors' yards. It looked so good. And that was because I have been going out there regularly and taking care of my yard.

How does this new behavior generator work? How does one break an old pattern, such as neglecting one's yard work and establish a new pattern? It is easy. Simply close your eyes and access your resourceful state of self-hypnosis. And in that resource state of self-hypnosis, focus on what you truly want to do, the yard looks as good as I possibly could, to make it stand out, to make it something I could be proud of. I envisioned in my mind the result of my efforts.

In my self-hypnosis, after creating a mental 8 x 10 glossy image of my yard being beautiful, I decided to expand that imagery into the scene of a movie. The kind of place where a Hollywood film scout might come and say, "We need a front yard of an average American neighborhood, and we'd love it if we could use your front yard." And so, I imagined my front yard is in a movie, and I imagined myself making a movie, a documentary of me taking care of my yard to make it good enough for a Hollywood movie. And thus, I created a movie in my mind of me trimming the hedges; I created a movie of me sweeping the walkways; I created a movie of me using the blower to remove debris from underneath the bushes in my yard.

I played these movie clips over and over, and gradually amplified the details of each—imagining the sound of the blower, the green of the well-watered leaves, the sound of me using the trimmers to trim the tree. All of these things were elements of my movie. I enjoyed playing that movie, and I amplified, and I paid attention to each of the attributes of me doing the work: I paid attention to the feeling of exercise—it's a good feeling; I paid attention to the feeling of sweat; I paid attention to the feeling of the sun and the vitamin D that was helping my body and my immune system become even stronger. I focused on all of the elements of putting together a complete cinematic compilation of the new behavior that I wanted to engage in.

What I did then is I put myself in three scenarios where I saw myself in that movie doing my yard work before a holiday weekend. I always appreciated in the past when my neighbors before the holiday weekend, Memorial Day, Labor Day, 4th of July, and Thanksgiving would make an effort to make their home look nice. So I pictured myself noticing an impending holiday on the calendar and getting ready to make my yard look nice. I then viewed myself in another scenario where yard work needed to be done after having rain during the rainy season when the yard can become dirty and muddy, and outside debris could be blown onto it. I saw myself cleaning up the mess that needed to be cleaned up following a storm, putting myself in that mental movie.

The third time, of course, is when the Hollywood producers came and said, "We'd like to feature your yard in a movie, make it look nice so that we can use it for a Hollywood movie shoot?" So, I pictured myself in that third scenario, getting ready to have my yard star in a Hollywood movie. And in self-hypnosis, I spent a day or two mentally rehearsing these scenes, these new behaviors in my mind. And guess what? The result has been that over the last several months, I've consistently had what I think is probably one of the best yards in the neighborhood. It was interesting. I was just out talking to my neighbor the other day, and he said, "Your yard always looks so nice." And I thought to myself, thank goodness I know the new behavior generator because I've set aside my old pattern of having the second-worst yard in the neighborhood and now I have the best in the neighborhood.

You can use this new behavior generator yourself. What behavior would you like to generate? Would you like to see yourself setting aside a portion of your paycheck each week and saving a hundred dollars in a savings account? Would you like to see yourself manicuring your nails rather than biting them? Would you like to see yourself responding with empathy and kindness rather than anger? This new behavior generator can be utilized literally with any behavior that you would like to create, but more importantly, that you would like to create an ongoing response.

The process is pretty simple: Close your eyes and create a mental picture, an 8 x 10 glossy photo, of the outcome that's important for you. See yourself in that image with the success that is important to you. Amplify that picture into a movie; it might only be a two or three-minute movie, perhaps a movie of you going through the drive-through window and depositing that paycheck but putting one hundred dollars into your savings account, and then coming home to log onto your online bank account and seeing your balance increase every week.

Next, create that mental movie, whatever it is, and amplify the aspects of the movie that make it real for you. Turn up the volume, make the color brighter, sharper, crisper, clearer. Pay attention to the aspects of it. Is the image far, or is the image near? Allow yourself to associate fully into this image and see yourself doing the tasks in this movie that are important to you. And then see yourself in three different scenarios, generating and using this new behavior. Taking a breath, allow yourself to feel awesome, knowing that what the mind can conceive, the body can achieve. Take in another breath. If your eyes aren't open, open them with a smile on your face, feeling fantastic, knowing that the new behavior generator is a powerful way for you to embrace success and to live your best life.

In the sample of saving money, see yourself saving money before purchasing something important. You have saved money over a long enough time, and the result is you can now create a better life for yourself doing the things that you want to do. In your movie, create a scenario where you are doing the task of saving money, and the result is something important or meaningful for you.

It's pretty cool to be able to create that new behavior and to see it in your mind. Perhaps the issue was getting a manicure and maintaining beautiful fingernails rather than biting them off. See yourself out for dinner, passing a plate, and somebody else noticing your beautiful nails. See yourself typing on your keyboard with your nails manicured and clean. See yourself in the third scenario, a third situation, where your nails are the way you would finally like them to be. Generate the new behavior of manicuring your nails and taking care of them regularly, rather than sporadically.

You can create an example, any scenario, any new behavior that would be useful to you. See yourself in three different scenarios or three different situations, manifesting that which you have created. And because we can use the creative mind to put ourselves into scenarios that we create, we can experience this in reality. Anything that exists in our physical world had to be a thought first.

You have generated this new behavior here in self-hypnosis. You have applied it in three different ways to three different scenarios. I do not doubt that by spending some time between now and next week, practicing the new behavior generator as an aspect of your self-hypnosis practice, you will discover that it is easy for you to manifest this, not only in the creative mind but in your real world as well.

CHAPTER 25:

Positive Thinking Meditation

Begin in a place you feel the most comfortable and relaxed. This area should be full of positivity.

Don't use a space where you will be distracted, stressed, or bombarded with negative thoughts. For example, avoid work or common areas where you feel tension or conflict with others. It should be a personal space that means something to you and where you won't feel fear or negativity creeping in.

You were keeping your legs straight out in front of you and arms hanging loosely by your side. If you are feeling stiff or too folded up, you won't be able to explore the positive energy coming into you.

Essential to have the right mindset in a mood where you are overcome or stuck on negative thinking from these thoughts and go into a place where you can healthily and happily start feeling more positive.

Notice your breath. Don't try to transform it in any way; simply feel as the air is coming into your body and as it leaves.

Start by breathing gently, and feel as your body fills with air. Allow this air to come out soft and delicately.

Don't breathe in any pattern yet. Just pay attention to how it naturally flows through you. Feel the fresh air come in, and the stale, warm air come out. You are breathing in good vibes.

You are breathing in happiness, positivity, and pure energy. You are breathing out evil thoughts and feelings that are weighing you down, keeping you stuck in the same toxic mindset.

Allow yourself to heal. Allow yourself to feel positive. It is okay to feel this way. Often, we don't like to stay positive because we might feel guilty. We might tell ourselves that it is not reasonable to remain positive when so many people in the world are angry, sad, and generally pessimistic.

That is not the way it has to be and perfectly acceptable for you to want to be happy. Just because other people might be living or thinking does not mean that you have to allow yourself to feel this same way.

Start to count your breath now. Focus your energy and make it easier to think positively. It's an exercise that you can apply whenever you need to change your pattern of thinking.

Breathe in. Count to five as you feel your lungs fill with air inside your body. As you breathe out, count down from five. Let this air come out slowly. Breathe in now for one, two, three, four, and five.

Breathe out now for five, four, three, two, and one. One more time, we are going to count down from ten. Breathe in for the first five and out for the last five. Continue this pattern as we finish throughout the meditation.

Changing how you think and noticing the one you have now. Let thoughts naturally pass through your mind now. Notice any that might be attached to negativity.

These thoughts are natural. Let them flow in and out as easily as you would any other part of your day. Except for this time, don't let the evil thoughts thrive, or even linger. Simply let it come into your mind and push it out with intention.

Pretend as though you are wading in a body of water, and the negative thoughts are like leaves or debris floating towards you. Each time a blade gets close, push it away gently with your hand. No need to pick it up or throw it. No need to push it away forcefully. Guide this thought away lightly with your fingers.

Each time you notice one of these negative thoughts, stop yourself, and turn it around. These thoughts are fears of what might happen tomorrow. Maybe you are afraid of going into work. Perhaps you are fearful of what somebody might think or do. Perhaps you are scared of a judgment call and making the wrong decision. Maybe it is a freak accident from the past that keeps you up at night. Each time you think of something like this, gently push it away.

Negative thoughts are also regretting that linger from the past. Maybe you are always thinking about what you should or could have done differently. Perhaps you are fearful of all the things that you missed, or you can't stop thinking about one decision you made a long time ago.

Each time one of these thoughts comes into your mind, push it out with tenderness. These thoughts aren't helping you. They aren't going to make you a more productive person. They're just going to keep holding you back. It is time to move forward.

We have to focus on the 'now.' The decisions that you've made cannot be changed. Everything that has already happened did so for a reason.

Notice your mindset and how you might be focusing only on the negative things. A dark and a light side to everything in our life. If you continuously stand in the dark, you will never be able to see all that is in the light.

Each time you have thoughts about what you do not have, remind yourself of all of the things that you do. A negative mindset is one that ignores all the chances for goodness. It is one that chooses not to see these aspects of life.

It is time to use gratitude. Gratitude is the appreciation of the things that you have in life. Both good and evil, you can find underlying recognition. It is not about being thankful for every single thing you have. You are merely noticing how these things have a positive impact on you.

Think of something terrible that has happened to you. What did you learn from this experience? What knowledge did you gain for the future? How were you able to go through this experience and still come out stronger because of it? These experiences are things that we can find benefits from, even if it was something horrible, we never wish to go through again.

There is still at least one lesson you can pull from it. Here we are just trying to find the diamond in the rough.

You are picking out that one small little beam of light through all the darkness. That does not make what happened okay, but it can help to change your mindset.

So, what lessons have you learned?

There is always something, albeit small, that is available to change your perspective for the better. It's up to you to find the gratitude in it. Continue to focus on your breathing as you notice these negative thoughts flowing away and creating a more positive mindset. Notice the negative thoughts slowing down. That makes it easier to focus on that positive energy and the bright light that beams down on your life.

Focus all of it on the good that you already have. Be ready to create more. Breathe in appreciation for everything that you have. Breathe out of any hate or anxiety you feel for the things that you don't have.

Breathe in joy and appreciation for all that surrounds us. Breathe out resentment and jealousy over people who seemingly have more than you. Breathe in the realization that you can get whatever you want. Breathe out the idea that you will be happy only when you have certain things.

Remember, we need to be incredibly appreciative of all that we have. Focus on this rather than focusing on all of the things that you still have to gain. One day, if you achieve all of these things, is that the only time that you are allowed to be happy? You should find a way to be positive all of the time. Don't limit the moments in which you show gratitude or appreciation.

You can be a happy individual at all times in life. You do not have to wait for good things to happen to feel or show happiness. You can do this at any moment. Breathe in the idea that it is okay to be happy. Breathe out any guilt you have over had a positive mindset.

There is no endpoint for happiness.

We were taught to keep a negative outlook, believing we are destined for misery, and only show appreciation for material things or monetary gains. We were instilled with thoughts that we are only allowed to be happy at the end of hard work. Struggle, reap the benefits, repeat. There is no time to focus on the past to interrupt this cycle.

You do not have to live like this. You can enjoy that struggle, and you can appreciate your time as you grow in life—no need to wait for the end to exhale and feel whole. You do not have to wait until you have everything that you've ever wanted to be happy. You are allowed to be happy right now.

Breathe in the idea that you are going to focus more on being happy now. Breathe out the idea that we have to have things to feel good. Evil doesn't always mean negative. Negative doesn't always mean bad. We can find appreciation from our greatest struggles. We can pull something of value out from all of the dust once it settles.

There will be struggles. Real-life is not one absent from challenge; an authentic experience is filled with gratitude, positivity, and appreciation for the problem—the chance to improve.

You are making a goal with yourself to do your best to power through any issue. Breathe in the idea that you're going to enjoy the journey. Breathe out the idea that you have to wait until the end of the turbulence to be happy.

Breathe in the idea that you are going to have a positive mindset throughout your entire journey. Breathe out the idea that you have to torture yourself and feel anguish over all of the challenges that you might have to endure. Focus on your breath once again. Notice as the air continues to come into your body, and how easily it leaves.

We can be grateful for this. We can have so much appreciation over the way that our bodies continue to breathe. How grateful are we that we can quickly fill our bodies with air and push it out without any effort! So many individuals are not able to breathe or move as we do. That is a small thing that we can start to understand and cherish. Think about this as you breathe in again. We're going to count down from ten. Breathe in for the first five and breathe out for the last five.

CHAPTER 26:

Affirmations for Losing Weight

Affirmations are statements made to amplify a particular idea. Affirmations are certainly going to help take you through your diet. You are going to want to repeat these affirmations when you are feeling both positive and negative. Whenever you feel like giving up or giving in, repeat these affirmations. Write them down, put notes around your home, and do whatever else is needed to keep you dedicated to your weight loss goals.

This first set of affirmations is going to be great if you are interested in working out and dieting to lose weight. These affirmations can be said while you are working out or while you are eating.

When you are working out, affirmations are going to be helpful to get you to a place where you don't want to give up. If you feel like you just want to throw in the towel, try some affirmations to keep you focused on what matters most—not giving up.

Sometimes, we might mindlessly eat as well. That can be dangerous because it means that we are not focused on eating healthy. That could end up leading to overeating or binge eating. If you want to control your portions, then these affirmations are helpful.

• I know that I have control over whether or not I will lose weight.

• I can get the body that I want.

• It is possible to achieve my dreams.

- I do not have to fantasize about my weight anymore. I have everything it takes to go through this process myself.

- I have no guilt over my past choices.

- Every decision I have made about my health has led me to where I am today.

- I am proud of my body that I have endured.

- I am grateful for the struggle that I have had with my body.

- The challenges I've faced with my health have helped me to be more appreciative of what I have.

- I might wish things were different with my body sometimes, but I know that I am grateful that they are the way they are now.

- I can do so much with my body.

- I know how to treat my body healthy so that I lose weight.

- I am losing weight all the time, not just at certain moments.

- As soon as I start to eat healthily, I feel lighter.

- Whenever I work out, I feel lighter.

- I am constantly losing weight, and it is making my body healthier.

- I know how to focus on healthy breathing.

- My breathing helps me to lose weight even more.

- When I am relaxed, I am happy.

- When I am happy, I am losing weight.

- I do not lose weight because I hate my body. I lose weight because I love my body.

- I am exercising to take care of my health.

- I am making healthy choices not just for me now, but for me later as well.

- I am reaching the weight that I want every day.

- I am continuously closer to getting the things that I have always wanted for my life.

- I am healing myself when I lose weight.

- My mind is improving just as much as my body is.

- I am blessed to have the mind and body that I have.

- I have important parts in my body that I need to be grateful for.

- My body could have less than what it has now, so I am grateful for the things that are present.

- I am focused on pushing through my exercises.

- Every time I want to give up exercising, I push forward because I know it will help me feel healthier.

- I make sure to eat something healthy instead.

- I do not torture my body with things that it cannot take.

- I am putting my body through the challenges needed to get the results that I want.

- I am focused on growing my body, not punishing it.

- I want to teach my healthy body habits, and that is what I am doing.

- I am helping my body be the best body possible.

- That is something that I deserve.

- I am working hard, and I deserve rewards.

- I am not hard on myself when I don't meet a goal that I was hoping for.

- I make sure to put myself first and keep moving on because I know that this is the most important thing that I can do.

- Believing in myself is what matters most.

- I know how to get the healthy body that I want, and there is nothing that is going to stop me.

- I am in charge of achieving my goals in life, and I am the one that is in charge.

Affirmations for Feeling Better

When we are feeling gross, ugly, or discouraged, then we are not feeling great. If you want to stick to a workout regime and lose weight, then you must emphasize feeling better. The better you feel, the easier it is going to be for you to have the confidence needed to make it to the gym, go for a walk, or attend the party.

Losing weight and getting healthy is important for you to feel better, not just to look better.

These affirmations are going to be useful for you to understand that as well.

Say these affirmations to yourself when you need to feel better, whether you are lazy or self-conscious.

Listen to these frequently, even every day, to help remind you that you deserve to look good but feel even better.

- I feel better and change myself based on the actions I choose to take.

- I have everything that I need to feel good.

- There is nothing that I can let make me feel bad at the moment.

- I have what it takes to feel good all the time.

- I am completely in control of my emotions.

- Others might do things that make me feel bad, but I am in control of how much I let these things affect me.

- I deserve to feel good in life.

- Others know that I deserve to feel good.

- Other people like being around me.

- Other people want me to feel good.

- I want others to feel good. We should all be feeling good.

- The positive attitude that helps me to feel even better.

- I am always excited and ready to start a new day.

- I look forward to what adventures might be waiting for me tomorrow.

- There is nothing in my life that scares me or holds me back from doing what I want.

- I have the confidence needed to accomplish my wildest dreams.

- I believe in myself, and that is what is going to power me through and help me find the things that I have been looking for.

- I have no problem deciding what I should do because I always know what is best.

- I know how to listen to my body, and I can tell whether it is feeling good or bad.

- I have so much joy that it overflows to others.

- I can spread how good I feel because I have so much positive energy.

- Even when I am in pain, it does not affect my mood.

- I appreciate the pain because I know it is presenting me with a healthy struggle.

- Everything that I will ever need is something that I already have.

- I don't have to be worried about anything making me feel bad because I have the power to change my perspective.

- I feel good and, therefore, I look good.

- I look good and, therefore, I feel good.

- There is nothing else I need to move forward to make me happy. Everything that does make me happy is going just to be an added benefit.

- I know what it takes to feel good.

- I make good decisions all the time so that I feel good all the time.

- I only include positive habits in my life that will help me to feel better overall.

- No one feels as good as I do.

- I care about how I feel because that is what matters first.

- I believe in myself, and that helps me to feel better.

- Whenever I am feeling down, I know how to turn my mood around and feel better.

- Everything that has happened bad in my life has taught me how to feel better.

- I am not afraid of what might be out there because I know that no matter how bad it might be, I will still be able to feel good.

- There are things I can't control in my life, but I know how to do what is important so that I am in control.

- I defeat challenges easily because I feel good about myself.

- I make sure to stand on what is right and fight for a good purpose.

- I always feel good because I choose to, even when things are tough.

- I know that feeling bad does me no good, so I will always focus on how I can feel good.

Conclusion

The more that you allow these types of exercises into your life, the more fit and active your mind will be. Having a healthy body is important, but if your mind isn't healthy first, it will be a much greater struggle.

This process requires willpower, strength, and discipline. Ensure that you can incorporate these into your life to see the results you've only been fantasizing about in the past. Pair this with other meditation books as well to get a variety of brain training that will keep you focused on your biggest dreams.

Your attitude can be one of those major things keeping you from reaching your fitness goals. Being on a healthy kick is not necessary for sustainable weight loss.

Losing weight is surely an amazing goal, but it is extremely hard to reach if there is no good motivation to encourage you to keep going.

It takes some time to reach that ideal weight, both time and effort, and to motivate yourself on this journey, and the best idea is to embrace positive self-talk.

You need to remind yourself of all of the amazing health benefits of losing weight, such as feeling more energized, feeling better about yourself, having a night of better sleep, and much more.

In addition to reminding yourself of all of the amazing health benefits of losing weight, another great idea is to keep a success journal where you will write every single step you have taken and succeeded in.

This way, you are more likely to stay committed to your weight loss journey. To boost your commitment, you also need to embrace some positive affirmations and positive self-talk, which will keep you going.

Therefore, the next time you look yourself in the mirror, instead of telling yourself I will never be thin and I will just give up, say to yourself this is going to be amazing, losing those five pounds feels great, and I will keep going.

Both of these statements are self-talk, but the first one is extremely negative self-talk, while the second one is positive self-talk.

These are automatic statements or thoughts to make to yourself consciously. Positive self-talk is an extremely important step as it can influence how you act or how you feel.

Instead of saying to yourself negative statements, embrace positive affirmations that come with some constructive ideas.

Once there, your positive self-talk can act as your guardian angel, destroying that annoying, destructive devil that has been sitting on your shoulder, keeping you from reaching your goals.

If you have battled to stay on the right track in the past, this is mostly due to that annoying negative self-talk, which, once there, brings failure, so you are more likely just to give up.

For this reason, say yes to positive self-talk. The most powerful thing about embracing positive self-talk is that those positive affirmations and positive statements you say to yourself tend to stick in your mind, so you are surrounded by positive feelings and thoughts.

CPSIA information can be obtained
at www.ICGtesting.com
Printed in the USA
BVHW041337081220
595180BV00006B/110